PSYCHOSOMATICS, PSYCHOANALYSIS, AND INFLAMMATORY DISEASE OF THE COLON

International Universities Press
Stress and Health Series

Edited by
Leo Goldberger, Ph.D.

Monograph 5

Psychosomatics, Psychoanalysis, and Inflammatory Disease of the Colon

Charles C. Hogan, M.D., D.Med.Sc.

International Universities Press, Inc.
Madison   Connecticut

Library of Congress Cataloging-in-Publication Data

Hogan, Charles C.
    Psychosomatics, psychoanalysis, and inflammatory disease of the colon / Charles C. Hogan.
       p. cm. — (Stress and health series : monograph 5)
    Includes bibliographical references and indexes.
    ISBN 0-8236-5732-9
    1. Inflammatory bowel diseases—Psychosomatic aspects.
    2. Psychoanalysis. I. Title. II. Series.
    [DNLM: 1. Inflammatory Bowel Diseases—psychology.
    2. Inflammatory Bowel Diseases—therapy. 3. Psychophysiologic
Disorders. 4. Psychoanalysis. W1 ST799K monograph 5 1994 / WI 420
H714p 1994]
RC862.I53H64 1995
616.3'44—dc20
DNLM/DLC
for Library of Congress   94-40750
                                                  CIP

Manufactured in the United States of America

TO MY WIFE, NINA,
whose love, help, editing and
typing made this book possible.

Contents

PART III PSYCHOANALYTIC TREATMENT

PART IV AFTERWORD

Acknowledgments

I want to express my appreciation to the founder of the Psychosomatic Discussion Group of the Psychoanalytic Association of New York, Inc., the late Dr. Melitta Sperling. She shared with us her many contributions to psychosomatic research and taught us the art and science of psychosomatic medicine. She chaired this group from 1960 until her death in 1973. Since that time the chairman has been Dr. C. Philip Wilson. I also want to extend my gratitude to the members of, and participants in, this organization: Drs. Leonard Barkin, Stephen L. Bennett, Sylvia Brody, Anna Burton, Lawrence Deutsch, H. Donald Dunton, Gerald Freiman, David Goldman, Eleanor Galenson, Henry Haberfeld, Jennifer Hunt, Cecelia Carol, Deborah S. Link, Charles McGann, Ira L. Mintz, Murial Gold Morris, Charles A. Sarnoff, Noah Shaw, Henry Schneer, Robert Schwartz, Christina Sekaer, Arthur Shore, Otto Sperling, Jacob Stump, and Barbara Wilson. Their help, support, and advice helped to make this book possible.

I am also indebted to other groups and academic institutions where material related to this volume has been presented in the forms of lectures, electives, symposia, or discussions. Among these are: The Psychosomatic Study Group of the American Psychoanalytic Association, chaired by Dr. C. Philip Wilson and cochaired by Dr. Howard Rudominer; the study group on Psychoanalytic Considerations About Patients with Organic Illness or Major Physical Handicaps of The American Psychoanalytic Association, chaired by Dr. Pietro Castelnuovo-Tedesco; the RAPS Group on Narcissism of The Association for Psychoanalytic Medicine chaired by Dr. Donald Meyers; my colleagues and students at The Albert Einstein College of Medicine, and the Chairman of the Department of Psychiatry, Dr. Toksoz Byram Karasu; my fellow faculty members and the candidates at The Columbia University Center for Psychoanalytic Training and Research under the directors the late Dr. John J. Weber, Dr. Ethel S. Person, and Dr. Roger A. MacKinnon; and my colleagues in The Association for Psychoanalytic Medicine.

I have been inspired and instructed by the contributors to the Melitta Sperling Memorial Lectures: Drs. Norman Atkins, Peter Blos, Jr., Lawrence Deutsch, Eleanor Galenson, James Herzog, Stanislav Kasl, Peter H. Knapp, Cecil Mushatt, George Pollock, Morton Reiser, Samuel Ritvo, Robert Savitt, Albert Solnit, Robert Tyson, and C. Philip Wilson.

There are special individual acknowledgments that I should like to add. First, I wish to thank Drs. C. Philip Wilson, Ira L. Mintz, and the late Dr. Cecil Mushatt for their help and encouragement as well as for their generous contributions to this volume. I am indebted for the encouragement, help, and advice of the late Dr. Lewis Fraad and Dr. Joel Katz who were generous enough to read and review some sections of this book. I have received immeasurable help with the bibliography from my daughter-in-law, Kristine Hogan. I wish to thank Dr. Margaret Emery, Dr. Leo Goldberger and International Universities Press for their editorial efforts.

And finally I want to express my admiration and gratitude for the hard work of my patients and the education that they afforded me as we mutually engaged in the long and usually rewarding tasks of psychoanalysis or psychoanalytic psychotherapy.

Foreword

Inflammatory disease of the colon has long been considered one of the most dramatic, treatment resistant, and potentially fatal of the psychosomatic diseases. Because the assumed causes of this illness span the broad spectrum from neurophysiological and genetic predisposition through unconscious conflict to familial and cultural factors, inflammatory disease of the colon raises fundamental theoretical questions regarding the interaction of biological and psychosocial determinants of illness.

Dr. Hogan has undertaken the challenging task of presenting a survey and study both of theories of psychosomatic disease in general and of Crohn's disease and ulcerative colitis in particular, in a book that can be read with profit by medical specialists, psychiatrists, and other mental health professionals. His historical review, presentation of the pathology, and detailing of the medical treatment are of particular interest, starting with Morgagni's clinical description of enterocolitis in 1769 in his celebrated *De Sedibus et Causis Morborum*.

After the brief historical summary, Dr. Hogan reviews the organic pathology and treatment of ulcerative colitis and Crohn's disease, including pharmaceutical, immunosuppressive, and surgical treatment that may result in symptom relief but are fraught with risks, potential side effects, and other complications. After an exploration of epidemiological, genetic, physiological, anatomical, and psychopathological considerations, Dr. Hogan turns his attention to an investigation of theories of psyche and soma, taking issue with other researchers and clinicians in the field on the issue of causality, emphasizing his agreement as a scientist with the proponents of the hypotheses of parallelism in the psyche and soma dispute. He buttresses his arguments with a discussion of linguistics, language, and the mind as an organization, and then proceeds to apply his ideas on parallelism to theories of conversion and the concept of stress. In his critique of alexithymia he shows that behind this defensive structure there is a world of primitive emotions, dreams, fantasies, archaic guilt, and magical thinking and he details the research that has culminated in theories of regulatory disturbances.

Drawing on thirty years of experience in the treatment of patients with psychosomatic disease as well as the supervision of professionals and the teaching of many courses in psychosomatics, Dr. Hogan explores the psychoanalytic treatment of diseases of the colon. Family background, parental psychopathology, object relations, fixations, and sexual development are detailed. Using ample clinical illustrations, he reviews the important early phase of treatment, the relation of the therapist to the medical specialist, and technical modifications such as the use of the couch. He then moves on into the most challenging and rewarding areas of psychodynamic research with these resistant patients: the technique of interpretation of primitive defensive positions, psychoses and transference psychoses, and the oedipal transference. A most important contribution for the psychoanalytic clinician is Dr. Hogan's chapter on countertransference, where he discusses denial and withdrawal, masochistic provocation, projective identification, and acting out.

This is a scholarly, exciting, and invaluable book by a master clinician who demonstrates that psychoanalysis and psychoanalytic therapy, by modifying the underlying personality disorder, can bring about the long-term resolution of inflammatory disease of the colon.

                                                    C. Philip Wilson, M.D.

Introduction

This volume discusses the successes that psychoanalysts have enjoyed in the treatment of inflammatory disease of the colon. The book includes studies of inflammatory gut disease from many points of view as well as a review and critique of psychosomatic concepts.

Its major contribution is the clinical evidence that psychoanalytic psychotherapy can reverse the course of inflammatory bowel disease. It is not unusual to see reversal proceed to a seemingly permanent remission or apparent "cure" of the physical symptoms. Above and beyond the medical results there are profound changes in the subjective worlds of our patients and the resolution of debilitating psychic conflicts.

I believe that inflammatory disease of the colon is the physical manifestation of a disorder that presents parallel physical and emotional manifestations. The goal of the psychoanalyst is to ameliorate or reverse the progress of both physical and psychic disorders, expecting a remission in both the physical and the parallel psychological symptomatology. This takes time, but with the help and support of teachers and colleagues who shared my interest in this work I reconfirmed the observations of many other psychoanalysts investigating psychosomatic diseases. I discovered that I could reach my goal in a reasonable percentage of cases, and I had a good idea of the reasons for failure when patients terminated without a resolution of their physical and mental problems. In my research of psychosomatic medicine, I tried to follow in the footsteps of Freud, Groddeck, Fenichel, F. Deutsch, Schur, Daniels, M. Sperling, O. Sperling,

Savitt, Mushatt and many other intuitive, capable, and creative psychoanalytic psychosomaticists.

There are a number of possible approaches to the treatment of inflammatory disease of the gut. The medical or surgical specialist attempts to ameliorate the physical symptoms through pharmaceutical or surgical intervention. The psychoanalytic physician has a profound interest in physical recovery, but his concerns encompass the resolution of the accompanying emotional conflicts. The clinical results are not considered a representation of a prolonged (perhaps life-long) remission until the accompanying emotional problems have been reasonably resolved and some symptom-free years have elapsed after the termination of treatment. Even patients who prematurely terminate treatment often enjoy an amelioration or termination of their physical symptoms.

My interest in the treatment of colonic disorders is part of my general interest in and long investigations in psychosomatic phenomenology and treatment. My early work in neurophysiology in Fredrick Mettler's laboratory at Columbia University's College of Physicians and Surgeons led to my doctoral work (Hogan, 1952) in the physiology of the caudate and anterior thalamic nuclei (Heath, Weber, Hogan, and Price, 1954) of the cat which interested me less than the research and reporting of the psychoanalytic pioneers in psychosomatic medicine. I then made a career decision that has been more than satisfying. Above and beyond teaching and supervision, I have practiced psychoanalysis and psychoanalytic therapy for forty years and have treated over 200 patients. From this series, I have selected those colitis patients described herein.

Part I is a general discussion of the historical, physical, epidemiological, genetic, and psychopathological aspects of ulcerative colitis and Crohn's disease of the colon. I review differential diagnoses, complications, and physical treatments including pharmacological (general as well as immunosuppressive) and surgical approaches.

In Part II I consider the sources and presentation of the scientific data that we record and communicate in our investigations of physical and emotional areas of a psychosomatic illness.

Of the many questions about observation and method floating around the worlds of linguistics, philosophy, and even medical literature, I like the linguist Whorf's observation (1941b): "For science's long and heroic effort to be strictly factual has at last brought it into entanglement with the unsuspected facts of the linguistic order. These facts the older classical science had never admitted, confronted, or understood as facts" (p. 246). Understanding linguistic rendition of data is important in all of science, but it takes on particular significance in our science, psychoanalysis, which requires the recovery of data from two sources: the subjective mind and the objective physical areas of observation.

I review a few of the approaches to, and models presented for, the study of psychosomatic medicine. I discuss linguistics and causality, and critically appraise the radical duality of entities in the common utilization of independence and interactionism. I present the philosophical concept of parallelism with isomorphism, Feigl's (1950, 1958) parallelism with dual language theory, Graham's (1967) paper on linguistic parallelism, and finally my own contribution on the acknowledgment of parallel sources of data.

I buttress my discussions with brief reviews of past and contemporary theories and definitions of causality. The noun-verb "cause" in medical thought and language is commonly used as a spatial metaphor instead of being assigned to its proper role in a temporal succession of events.

I conclude this section with a discussion of how linguistic understanding of clinical data affects our understanding of conversion, stress, alexithymia, and self-regulatory concepts of psychoanalysis. Part II, in sum, directs the reader's attention to important work in medicine, philosophy, and linguistics that can help clarify the mind–body problem.

In Part III, Psychoanalytic Treatment, I return to clinical data and discuss psychoanalysis and psychoanalytic psychotherapy of patients with inflammatory disease of the colon. After an historical review of the literature on the psychoanalytic treatment of inflammatory gut disease, I explore the content and dynamics of its psychopathology, followed by a discussion of technical considerations. The concluding chapters discuss transference and countertransference. Throughout are, I hope, sufficient details about the problems and conflicts observed in the mental life of colitis patients so that the uninitiated psychoanalytic traveler can know a little of the country to which he may wish to journey.

I have two hopes: the first is to stimulate psychoanalytic interest in the individual with inflammatory bowel disease, the second to contribute to a broader and deeper understanding of how an observer of a psychosomatic disease works with parallel (dual) sets of data, and reports that data in parallel linguistic styles.

Part I
What Is and Is Not Inflammatory Disease of the Colon?

Chapter 1
Brief Historical Review

Throughout written history there have been documentary and fictional allusions to every conceivable variety of intestinal disease and discomfort. Constipation, diarrhea, fecal incontinence, intestinal hemorrhage, prolapse, and innumerable other medical complications of the large and small intestine have found their way into the world's literature, where these disabilities have not infrequently been directly linked in one way or another to emotional conflicts. Gut activity has been presented in terms of the subjective perceptions of the victim and described from the somewhat detached parallel position of an observer. Medications, surgical procedures, and emotional manipulations have been alternatively recommended and reviled as either nostrums for or initiators of disease.

The first known clinical description of enterocolitis with particular involvement of the colon was contributed by Morgagni in *De Sedibus et Causis Morborum* (The Seats and Causes of Disease) (1769).

Much of the early investigative reporting on bowel inflammation came from Guy's Hospital in London where Samuel Wilks (1859a) first referred to inflammatory processes in the colon in his lecture on pathological anatomy. That same year (1859b) he testified in court on the pathological findings in the colon of a young woman. In this testimony he presented a classical description of the histopathology of ulcerative colitis.

Wilks along with Walter Moxon (Wilks and Moxon, 1875, pp. 408–409) gave a series of lectures on pathological anatomy, again referring to a number of cases in which death and the

3

pathological findings in the gut were consistent with inflammatory bowel disease. Each death had followed a long-standing debilitating illness.

Allchin (1885) reported on a case of extensive ulceration of the colon in a young woman admitted to Westminster Hospital in London.

White (1888) reviewed the pathological findings in a series of inflamed colons in autopsied cases from Guy's Hospital. The assumed cause of death was the colonic pathology. As one reviews his descriptions, it seems apparent that Crohn's disease as well as ulcerative colitis were probably present in the specimens observed. Ileitis was present in varying degrees in cases 2, 4, 9, 10, and 11 of the eleven reported postmortems.

Dalziel (1913) of Glasgow gave excellent descriptions of nine patients with ileitis characterized by granulomatous lesions that he first suspected of being tubercular. This would be of only indirect interest to us except for the intimate association (and/or identity) of this ileitis with the later described Crohn's disease. Over the next two decades there were a great many reports of ulcerative colitis as well as ileitis, but our knowledge of the physical pathology of these groups of illnesses was substantially broadened in 1932. At that time, Crohn, Ginzburg and Oppenheimer described a disease of the terminal ileum in young adults (1932, p. 1324) with a granulomatous pattern and with a marked tendency toward perforation and fistulae formation. Since these observations, cases such as those described by Dalziel (1913) and later by Crohn (1932) have collectively been known as Crohn's ileitis.

The granulomatous histopathology that characterizes this disease was soon found in the colon as well as other portions of the gastrointestinal tract. Lockart-Mummery and Morson (1960) distinguished pathology in the colon similar to that described in 1932 by Crohn et al. from what they felt was a separate disease entity, ulcerative colitis.

Atwell, Duthie, and Coligher (1965, p. 970) noted that Crohn's disease may affect any part of the alimentary tract from the esophagus to the anal canal. Bruno (1979) has commented that "anal symptoms are often the presenting problem [of Crohn's] and the true incidence of anorectal Crohn's disease is something that has only recently been documented" (p. 7; see chapter 2).

The investigation of psychic conflict associated with inflammatory bowel disease really began with the observations of Cecil Murray (1930a,b; see chapter 12).

Freud (1895, pp. 95 and 98) was the first to make a connection between diarrhea and constipation and 'psychic conflict. Sandor Ferenczi (1919, pp. 89–104) discussed the discreet conscious and unconscious control that the mind can exert on the activity of the gut. Karl Abraham (1920, pp. 318–322; 1921, pp. 370–392; 1924, pp. 425–428) devoted a great deal of attention to psychic control of the gut. However, none dealt directly with inflammatory disease of the colon.

Chapter 2
Organic Pathology and Treatment

A psychoanalytic physician interested in a psychological approach to the problems of inflammatory bowel disease should be familiar with the anatomy, organic pathology, and histopathology of these processes. He or she should also have a thorough knowledge of other pertinent data such as epidemiology, prognosis, medical treatment, surgical treatment, and possible complications of the disease or of the treatment procedures. A physician who anticipates treatment of these conditions from a psychoanalytic perspective needs to be more than just familiar with these factors. He or she should be academically and clinically acquainted with these diseases through supervised experience in the psychoanalytic treatment of patients with inflammatory bowel disease.

Anatomically, inflammatory bowel disease can involve any or all layers: the mucosa, the submucosa, the muscularis, and the serosa as well as the peritoneal surfaces and the lymphoid tissues of the colon. It appears to be an idiopathic inflammatory process that does not involve bacterial, viral, or physically traumatic factors. The small intestine may be involved, more so in Crohn's disease, which may, in fact, be limited to ileitis. Ileocolonic involvement can occur with either Crohn's disease or ulcerative colitis. However, here we will limit our discussion to pathological processes in the colon, because the clinical experience of the author, and most other psychoanalytic investigators, has been concerned primarily with this organ.

7

Earlier cases were grouped together as inflammations of the intestinal tract. As noted in the previous chapter, Crohn, Ginzburg, and Oppenheimer (1932) first described a disease of the terminal ileum in young adults which pathologically displayed a granulomatous pattern and showed a marked tendency toward perforation (p. 1324). The same pathological picture was discovered in the colon and Atwell, Duthie, and Coligher (1965) observed that this granulomatous process could involve every part of the "alimentary tract from the esophagus to the anal canal" (p. 970).

While there are many similarities between ulcerative colitis and Crohn's disease of the colon, a number of gross and histopathological differences have been described and documented. There are also some very important differences in the manner in which each of these entities responds to pharmaceutical and surgical treatment.

I anticipate later discussion of psychological similarities and differences by noting here that McKegney, Gordon, and Levine (1970) in an extensive study of patients with ulcerative colitis and Crohn's disease observed: "There are no significant differences between the patients with the two diseases in a large number of demographic, psychosocial, personality, behavioral, psychiatric, and physical disease characteristics. *In both syndromes, more severe emotional disturbance is associated with more severe demonstrable physical disease*" (p. 153; emphasis added).

It is also worthy of note that Cook and Dixon (1973) wrote:

> There is a range of appearances in inflammatory diseases of the colon which form a continuous spectrum, the ends of which are easily labelled as either ulcerative colitis or Crohn's disease. Between these extremes any given feature may vary in frequency or severity and independently of the other pathological changes. This results in an infinite number of pathological appearances and great difficulty in separating the diseases into pathological entities.
>
> The great need is for pathologists to describe cases in detail without clinical opinion prejudicing their reporting and to concentrate less on forcing the case before them into a largely clinically defined category (pp. 259–260).

Fawaz, Glotzer, Goldman, Dickersin, Gross, and Patterson (1976) indicated that the diagnosis of one or the other clinical entity must be based on a multifactorial analysis, observations to be kept in mind as we attempt to describe the similarities and differences in what may appear to be two separate disease processes. Cook and Dixon (1973) seem to infer the probability of a continuum between these two pathological processes.

ULCERATIVE COLITIS AS A PHYSICAL ENTITY

Bruno's (1979) description of the gross anatomical lesions in ulcerative colitis is worth quoting:

> Ulcerative colitis is a confluent, erosive, inflammatory process which is symmetrical and specifically involves the mucosal surfaces of the colon. It may occasionally extend beyond the mucosa to involve the submucosa, but it is basically a mucosal disease. It most commonly involves the rectum, rectosigmoid and left colon. In many of the cases, the distribution of the disease process stops abruptly at the midtransverse colon for reasons that are not apparent. Approximately 30% of these patients have total involvement of the colon; half of this group also have involvement of the terminal ileum. When that is the case, radiographic differentiation from Crohn's disease may be difficult. The most common distribution of ulcerative colitis, of course, is ulcerative proctitis. . . . ulcerative colitis is basically a symmetrical confluent mucosal disease. . . . The mucosa is confluently ulcerated with residual mucosal bridges: sometimes there is complete effacement of the mucosa. Pseudopolyps are an important pathological feature of this disease, due to hypertrophy of some of the residual islets of colonic mucosa [p. 6].

Măratka (1986) notes that evaluation of the microscopic features may be difficult because most specimens come from advanced cases. He makes clear that in ulcerative colitis "the initial change is in the mucosa and is characterized by *haemorrhagicocatarrhal inflammation* with crypt abscesses and goblet cell depletion" (p. 33).

Cook and Dixon (1973) summarized their studies and observations: "The features which have been shown to be most accurate and valuable in the diagnosis of ulcerative colitis include a 'healed granular' mucosa, a continuous inflammatory pattern, an irregular gland pattern, and the absence of fissures" (p. 255).

Occasionally, one encounters fistulae and/or abscesses, usually in the anal rectal area, described below under complications. However, these complications are not common throughout the gut as they are in Crohn's disease. The infrequently occurring fistulae in ulcerative colitis are most commonly seen perianally.

In short, we may note that while in some instances there may be isolated involvement of submucosal tissues, ulcerative colitis is a symmetrical confluent mucosal disease (Bruno, 1979, p. 6).

INITIATING SYMPTOMS OF ULCERATIVE COLITIS

The initiating symptoms of ulcerative colitis vary according to author. Engel (1954a) first called attention to the prominence of bleeding (p. 417) as an initiating symptom as opposed to diarrhea which had previously been emphasized. In the same paper he noted (p. 417) that chronic constipation is sometimes a symptom and may occasionally be the presenting symptom. Of course, bloody diarrhea and/or abdominal pain or cramps are common early problems, as we might expect from our knowledge of the pathological anatomy of the disease process. Engel (1956) also called attention to the high percentage of ulcerative colitis patients who had a history of severe and persistent headaches prior to the initiation of the intestinal illness as well as during the disease process (p. 334.)

There are on occasion some unusual presenting symptoms. Castelnuovo-Tedesco (1966) described a case in which gout preceded the onset of ulcerative colitis. I treated a patient who suffered from recurrent eczema which disappeared after the onset of ulcerative colitis, but which reappeared during early remissions while the patient was in psychoanalytic treatment. A second patient had occasional recurrent eczema while in treatment, but this was not an initiating symptom (Hogan, 1989).

I have no doubt that there are numerous individual variations, but the usual noticeable early symptoms are blood, diarrhea, and/or abdominal cramping. We shall see that this somewhat dramatic colon symptomatology in ulcerative colitis may differ from the initiating symptoms of Crohn's disease (particularly Crohn's ileitis).

COMPLICATIONS

The serious complications of ulcerative colitis are numerous and may involve almost any of the body's systems, intestinal or extraintestinal. The variety of symptomatic accompaniments was very well summarized by Sidaron (1986), and I shall mention a few here.

Intestinal complications: One of the most important on a long-term basis is carcinoma of the colon described by Crohn and Rosenberg (1925), Goldgraber, Humphreys, Kirsner, and Palmer (1958, 1959), Goldgraber and Kirsner (1964), Kirsner and Shorter (1975, 1980, 1988), Goodman and Sparburg (1978), among many others. Goldgraber and Kirsner noted (1964) that frequency varied ranging from 0.6 percent to 14 percent. Lightdale and Sherlock (1988) feel that the incidence is less than 2 percent during the first ten years of the illness and may be less in office practice than in patients who have been hospitalized (p. 282).

Other intestinal complications are toxic megacolon, strictures, perforation, peritonitis with or without perforation, pseudopolyposis, abscess formation (often perianal), hemorrhage and exsanguination.

Occasional fissures and fistulae may form with ulcerative colitis, particularly in the anal rectal area, but they are very rare elsewhere in the gastrointestinal tract. They are exceedingly common throughout the intestinal tract in Crohn's disease.

Extraintestinal complications can touch almost every bodily system. Joints may be involved in complications such as ankylosing spondylitis, sacroilietis, or peripheral arthritis.

The skin may show erythema nodosom, pyoderma gangrenosum, epidermolysis, bulla acquisita (Raab, Fretzin, Bronson, Scott, Roenak, and Medenica, 1983), lichen planus, and so forth. As noted earlier, I have observed eczematoid rashes occurring during remissions in the illness while patients were under psychoanalytic treatment (Hogan, 1989).

The eyes may suffer with conjunctivitis, keratitis, episclerites, corneal ulceration, anterior uveitis, optic nerve obliteration, or blephoritis. Stomatitis and ulcerations of the mouth are not uncommon.

In the liver we may occasionally find pericholangitis, hepatic steatosis, sclerosing cholangitis, chronic active hepatitis, or cirrhosis. The cardiovascular system may give evidence of pericarditis, myocarditis, vasculitis, giant cell arteritis, venous thrombosis, or anemia.

Engel (1956) noted the high incidence of headaches, both tension and migraine, during and preceding the illness. I have discussed typical migraine headaches which first appeared during the psychoanalytic treatment of a patient with ulcerative colitis (Hogan, 1989). They disappeared as certain conflicts were analyzed and have not reappeared during the prolonged remission of illness following termination.

PROGNOSIS

Prognostic evaluations differ from author to author. Here I refer to Goodman and Sparberg (1978). There seems to be a mortality rate with a severe attack of 5 percent to 10 percent; with a moderate attack, 1 percent to 2 percent; and virtually 0 percent in mild attacks. There is an annual death rate of 1 percent in patients under 60 and 5 percent in patients over 60. In young adults the 20-year survival rate is 95 percent of the expected rate (p. 190). "It seems that ulcerative colitis always relapses eventually" (Goodman and Sparberg, 1978, p. 151).

PHARMACEUTICAL TREATMENT

Medical treatment with drugs (Hanauer and Kirsner, 1989) may include the usual palliative medications such as antispasmotics or opiates, particularly in the early treatment of an uncomplicated illness.

Since 1950, when corticosteroids were first used at the Mayo Clinic to treat ulcerative colitis, they have played an important role in the treatment of inflammatory bowel disease. As Babb (1988a) stated:

> Experimentally, they [steroids] reduce capillary permeability, inhibit the migration of leukocytes and macrophages into inflamed areas, block T cell response to antigens and macrophage activation, impair the ability of leukocytes to release proteolytic enzymes and decrease prostoglandin and leukotriene production. Moreover, in the normal and inflamed colon they increase sodium and water transport from lumen into the lining cells, thereby decreasing diarrhea. Thus the use of corticosteroids in the treatment of patients with ulcerative colitis, a disease characterized by signs and symptoms of inflammation, is rational [p. 365].

Steroids have been used in virtually every form by almost every avenue of administration: oral, enema, suppository, intramuscular, and intravenous routes. As to their ultimate efficacy, they seem to terminate acute exacerbations in severe ulcerative colitis in 40 to 55 percent of patients within one or two weeks, and in moderately severe colitis at a rate of 60 percent to 80 percent of patients reported Babb (1988a), who notes that there are questions about the preferred route of administration and dosage of the various steroids. "Therapeutic decisions are currently based on bias, past training, and ongoing experience" (p. 366).

Another treatment that at times helps ameliorate or terminate an acute exacerbation of ulcerative colitis is sulfasalazine. It is a matter of interest that, unlike the steroids, this group of compounds is not usually utilized in the treatment of Crohn's disease.

Sulfasalazine (salicylazosulfapyradine), known as Azopyrin, and Azulfidine is usually administered by mouth and seems to shorten the length of exacerbations. Because it is not absorbed in the small intestine, 90 percent reaches the colon where it is split by intestinal bacteria into evidently inactive sulfapyradine and 5-amino salicylic acid, which seems to be the active ingredient absorbed in the colon. 5-amino salicylic acid is absorbed in the small intestine if it is not in the chemical compound with sulfapyradine, which for the most part is excreted from the colon. Several attempts have been made to synthesize compounds that utilize 5-amino salicylic acid in the colon, avoiding its absorption in the small intestine, without the wasted sulfapyradine.

Lauritsen, Laursen, Bukhave, and Rask-Madsen (1987, p. 166) called attention to the frequency of exacerbations with the withdrawal of sulfasalazine and talked of the possibility of continuing administration through remissions. But we do not know how sulfasalazine acts on the colon. Such drugs may or may not be combined with one of the steroid anti-inflammatory drugs such as ACTH or prednisone either by mouth, suppository, or enema. Lauritsen et al. (1987, p. 166) noted that nonsteroidal anti-inflammatory drugs are without clinical efficacy, and may even worsen active disease.

Hyperalimentation, often by total parenteral nutrition, blood transfusions, and other more radical forms of medical intervention are occasionally used in severe cases of ulcerative colitis.

Karush, Daniels, Flood, and O'Connor (1977) compared patients treated in the years before the advent of steroid treatment (as supportive medical treatment) with our contemporary patients who receive steroids or steroids and Azulfidine. "Supportive treatment" refers to the traditional care used before the advent of steroids. Karush et al. concluded:

1. More than half of patients undergoing supportive medical treatment for ulcerative colitis will enter remission within six months [Those patients not receiving steroids or sulfasalazine].
2. The cumulative six month remission rate is roughly the same with supportive therapy as with steroid therapy.
3. Steroid therapy induces a remission more rapidly in a large number of cases.
4. The relapse rate for patients undergoing supportive medical treatment was lower than for the steroid treated group.
5. In a group of patients with atypical colitis [Crohn's disease], the remission and relapse rate were very similar to those for typical ulcerative colitis.
6. The presence of ileal disease results in a lower six-month remission rate with supportive treatment. With steroid therapy, the remission rate is nearly the same as when there is no ileal involvement [p. 21].

With our present medical treatment modalities, particularly the steroids, the length of exacerbations has been reduced in some cases, but there is some question as to the effect on long-term outcome. As Korelitz and Gribetz (1962) noted: "The number of complications of ulcerative colitis in steroid treated patients has not been obviously reduced" (p. 576).

Goodman and Sparberg (1978) concluded that:

Corticosteroids can be used systemically (parenterally or orally) or topically in the rectum. They are effective in suppressing an attack of the disease and in inducing a remission that usually, but by no means always persists after they are withdrawn. Their long term use is fraught with side effects and has been shown by Trulove to be ineffective in preventing relapse of quiescent disease [p. 110].

Patients on prolonged steroid therapy show the usual signs of toxicity such as osteoporosis. Children and adolescents are prone to developmental defects, particularly in rates of growth and size. Sperling (1969) noted:

Follow-up study of thirty-seven children aged two and a half to eleven and a half years, treated with steroids during the first three years of the disease, later revealed an even higher incidence of chronic complications compared with the results in the presteroid era, and a higher frequency of retarded growth and development, possibly accentuated by direct hormonal influence . . . treatment has not reduced the incidence of surgery [p. 337].

Sperling was quoting Korelitz and Gribetz (1962), who also concluded that "the number of complications of ulcerative colitis in the steroid treated patients has not been obviously reduced" (p. 596).

In the research area, literally thousands of studies involving single drugs or combinations in various ratios and dosages have been done in the last 40 years.

IMMUNOSUPPRESSIVE DRUGS

Since 1962 there have been a number of studies of the treatment of ulcerative colitis with immunosuppressive agents, which yielded gratifying short-term results, albeit with some severe complications. This material was extensively reviewed in 1989 by Daniel H. Present.

Bean was the first to use 6-Mercaptopurine with one case in 1962. He reported successful results and followed up with a 1966 study. Despite feeling his results were close to miraculous, he noted relapses if the drug was stopped. Winkelman and Brown (1965) used nitrogen mustard in the treatment of chronic ulcerative colitis and regional enteritis. They reported dramatically gratifying short-term results, but also noted the toxicity of the drug and the large number of severe complications. Bowen, Irons, and Rhodes (1966) first used azathioprine with ulcerative colitis patients; in 1984 Gupta, Keshavazian, and Hodgson reported the use of cyclosporin.

One should note that in most, but not in all cases steroids are continued with the use of immunosuppressive drugs. One of the advantages claimed for such drugs is the reduction of other medications. Present, whose experience was with 6-Mercaptopurine, summarized his and Korelitz's experiences with one series of sixty patients (1989):

> The response rate in refractory patients is 73 per cent (43 per cent complete remission and 30 per cent moderate improvement). . . . As with Crohn's disease, the onset of action is also slow (mean of 3 months) and steroids can be discontinued or lowered in close to 70 per cent of patients. . . . the drug does not appear to be as effective in maintaining a remission once this has been induced [p. 65].

However he also states that "the drug should be maintained for approximately 2 to 3 years after induction of remission" (p. 69).

Present, Meltzer, Krumholtz, Wolke, and Korelitz (1989) reported on the toxicity of 6-Mercaptopurine over an 18-year period with 396 ulcerative colitis and Crohn's disease patients. Their summary noted that "follow up data for a mean period of 50.3 months were obtained for 90% of the patients." They found pancreatitis, 3.3 percent; bone marrow depression, 2 percent; allergic reactions, 2 percent; drug hepatitis, 0.3 percent.

> Infectious complications were seen in 29 patients (7.4%), of which 7 (1.8%) were severe, including one instance of herpes zoster encephalitis. All infections were reversible with no deaths. Twelve neoplasms (3.1%) were observed, but only one (0.3%), a diffuse histiocytic lymphoma of the brain, had a probable association with the use of 6-mercaptopurine [p. 641].

Immunosuppressive drugs are associated with a high rate of neoplasia in transplant patients. Lymphoma is the most common neoplastic complication (Present, 1989, p. 67).

While short-term results with immunosuppressive drugs does seem to hold promise in the realm of pharmaceutical treatment, one can see that their use is not without risk. The really long-term therapeutic results are not yet in, particularly in terms of long-term, drug-free remission. The long-term results on toxicity also await an eventual evaluation.

PHARMACEUTICAL EVALUATION

Results of pharmaceutical intervention should be compared to the long-range drug-free results in patients who have received intensive psychoanalytic psychotherapy (see chapter 12). Even though the organic symptoms may be held in check with drugs in some patients, severe accompanying characterological psychopathology remains untreated.

Although there is a plethora of investigations into the gross-pathological, histopathological, neurophysiological, biochemical, and immunological aspects of ulcerative colitis, it is not my immediate interest, nor is it possible, to even approach either a summary or an indication of the breadth of the research involved; all of which touch upon the possibility of improvement in the pharmaceutical treatment of the organic symptoms of this disease. At this moment, however, pharmaceutical treatment leaves much to be desired.

SURGERY

Surgical intervention, in the form of colectomy and ileostomy, is often seen as an important life-saving measure in ulcerative colitis. It has even been recommended as a prophylaxis against carcinoma. Surgery has been utilized whenever there is any doubt about possible complications. Surgery is viewed with much greater reservation in Crohn's disease of the colon than it usually is in ulcerative colitis.

Even the best of surgical procedures carry with them a certain risk. Goodman and Sparberg (1978) note that the operative mortality of a total colectomy when performed as an emergency procedure is roughly 15 percent to 30 percent; elective colectomy is 2 percent or less; between 10 percent and 20 percent of patients with permanent ileostomy will need further surgery.

Block and Shraut (1988) listed the complications of surgery with colectomy, including all of the usual possibilities in gut surgery such as infection, wound separation, incidental hernia, generalized peritonitis, peritoneal sepsis, or abscesses. They noted that 14 percent of ordinary ileostomies required revision of the stoma within ten years.

The psychological effects of and responses to social activities are immense, particularly in younger people. Attempts to ameliorate the often devastating effects of the surgery are constantly evolving. The success of modifications in surgical procedures have been far better in ulcerative colitis than in Crohn's disease.

Surgical approaches to the colon in both ulcerative colitis and Crohn's disease of the large bowel usually involve total colectomy with the resultant ileostomy requiring an external receptacle for fecal retention. (Occasionally partial colectomy and even more occasionally colorectal anastomosis were performed in the past, but until recently, such procedures were the exceptions.) The hope with recent surgical modifications is that traditional ileostomy can be replaced with some sort of internal reconstruction allowing at least a measure of personal control over the time and place of the disposal of fecal material.

Newer surgical procedures still involve removal of all or part of the colon, but attempts are made to construct either anal anastomosis or cathetar openings. Such proceedures have given a measure of help and confidence to many patients after a period of adjustment. Most patients prefer one of the newer reconstructions to the old open ileostomy.

Some of the newer surgical procedures are described by Dozois and Kelly (1988). One is the removal of the caecum, colon, and proximal rectum. Only the mucosa is removed from the distal colon and/or rectum. The ileorectal anastomosis in many cases preserves voluntary transanal defecation and usually helps preserve some fecal continence. This surgery is at times combined with the construction of an ileal pouch as described below.

Another approach is a continent reservoir ileostomy (Dozois and Kelly, 1988, p. 667) in which an ileal pouch is constructed that collects and stores ileal effluent. A valve that makes the pouch continent for gas and feces is constructed with a conduit leading to the stoma. The patient maintains continence until a catheter is inserted through the stoma.

There are complications (Ruderman, 1987; Petras, Bona, McGonagle, and Fazio, 1987). A new illness, "pouchitis," has been discovered—a form of ileitis that occurs in pouches whether constructed surgically for ulcerative colitis or family polyposis. Ruderman lists the complications of pouch construction in continence preserving reservoirs as: pouch obstructions, 39 percent; mesh erosion, 13 percent; peripouch abscesses, 11 percent; Crohn's disease, 5 percent; and finally, pouchitis, 23 percent.

Even with the best of procedures, the quality of life changes. Unfortunately, patients often decline opportunities to voice the intensity of their fears, complaints, and shame unless given the possibility of recognizing their defenses against such admissions. Their reluctance is of particular importance in patients with inflammatory disease of the bowel who are inclined to use denial and suppression to an unusual degree. Many are terrified at the idea of exposing loss of control or helplessness (see chapters 11 and 13). Patients' brief responses to brief questions about their altered life patterns are often, if not usually, quite different from the associations that analysts hear in their daily sessions where patients, over time, are able to express themselves freely and spontaneously, without shame or the fear of hurting someone else's feelings. At best the altered life-style is anything but pleasant and is not a desirable way to solve a problem if any alternative to an ileostomy is available.

As a final note in the description of ulcerative colitis, the onset and progression of ulcerative colitis tends to be less severe when it appears in the older age group. Conversely, as M. Sperling (1978b) noted, "the course of this illness in children is more severe than in adults and the response to medical treatment is less satisfactory. The earlier the onset of ulcerative colitis, the more severe will be its course" (p. 62).

In my very brief overview of the anatomical aspects of ulcerative colitis, I trust that I have demonstrated the serious nature of the disease and some of the specific physical problems involved. To most patients the pain, discomfort, and possible related disabilities of the disease and treatment are of major concern and impose serious interferences with the rhythm of normal life. The symptoms of ulcerative colitis can be catastrophic.

In the following section, I shall discuss the other inflammatory disease of the colon that seems related to the, sometimes more benign, ulcerative colitis. I want here to call attention to the work of Cook and Dixon (1973, p. 259) in which they infer the probability of a continuum in their observations of the histopathological changes in these two diseases.

CROHN'S DISEASE OF THE COLON AS A PHYSICAL ENTITY

Granulomatous colitis or Crohn's disease was originally described as an inflammatory process involving only the terminal ileum (Crohn et al., 1932). As noted by Atwell et al. (1965, p. 970), it is now recognized as a disease that involves any segment of the gastrointestinal tract.

For a brief summary of the clinical pathology of this entity, I again begin with Bruno (1979). Crohn's ileocolitis "is the most common form of the disease and it is more common than the disease restricted to the terminal ileum. It is important to emphasize that anal symptoms are often the presenting problem and the true incidence of anorectal Crohn's disease is something that only recently has been documented" (p. 7).

As has been presented by Crohn et al. (1932) and Lockhart-Mummery and Morson (1960), the inflammatory process in Crohn's disease involves all of the layers of the intestine, often including the peritoneal. It is submucosal. Granulomata and microgranulomata are common.

Bruno (1979) says: "Transverse fissuring and lymphoid hyperplasia and lymphangiectasia, and crypt abscesses containing eosinophils and macrophages are not uncommon" (p. 7).

As Cook and Dixon (1973) summarized their studies and observations: "The features that have been found to be most accurately observed in the diagnosis of Crohn's disease include confluent linear ulcers, deep fissures, an aggravated inflammatory pattern and sarcoid like granulomata" (p. 253).

Măratka (1986) emphasizes that the "initial lesion in CD [Crohn's disease] is in the *lymphoid follicles* and *Peyer's patches* of the mucous membrane which undergo hyperplasia followed by ulceration. In this way 'aphthoid ulcers' originate, which are the typical feature of early CD. . . . CD is essentially a disorder of the lymphoid tissue of the gastrointestinal tract" (p. 33).

There may be peritoneal involvement, and thus fistulous tract formation is extremely common. As Bruno (1979) observed, "[it] is one of the most devastating features of this process" (p. 8).

Skip areas of involvement are not unusual. Stricture formation and obstruction are far more frequent in Crohn's disease than in ulcerative colitis.

To summarize, Crohn's disease of the colon is usually a noncontiguous process that involves all layers of the large bowel. Often it is of a severe inflammatory nature and is frequently characterized by fistulae, fissures, and strictures.

INITIATING SYMPTOMS

Initiating symptoms are often less obvious and less dramatic than those presented by many ulcerative colitis patients. Anorexia, weight loss, and fever of unknown origin are frequently the first symptoms. Some cases in adolescent female patients have been misdiagnosed as anorexia nervosa. Developmental defects and nutritional difficulties are not unusual. Persistent nonbloody diarrhea can be present. Malaise and abdominal cramping may accompany other symptoms.

If the disease involves the anal–rectal area, symptoms similar to ulcerative colitis, including bloody diarrhea, may be present.

COMPLICATIONS

The serious and chronic complications of Crohn's disease are often the same as those of ulcerative colitis, including the increased vulnerability to carcinoma of the gastrointestinal tract. I observe below that the areas of involvement are often different from those in ulcerative colitis.

As I have noted, the one important exception is the tendency toward fistulae formation, particularly as the disease progresses, and may involve almost any part of the gastrointestinal tract (Korelitz, 1979). Fistulae may be ileocolonic, colon-bladder, ileo- or colon-peritoneal. They may invade the peritoneum and penetrate the muscular walls of the abdominal cavity. This gives rise to epitheleal or mucous membrane involvement leading to draining fistulae on the abdomen, on the perineum, or in the vagina.

The tendency toward stricture formation may cause exceedingly painful symptoms, particularly if the Crohn's is in the rectal–anal region.

Perforation is much more common in Crohn's than in ulcerative colitis, as is intra-abdominal abscess formation. Pseudopolyposis is far less common in Crohn's than in ulcerative colitis (Huizenga and Schroeder, 1988, p. 258).

Associated nutritional deficiencies are almost universal, including deficits in protein, zinc, magnesium, vitamin B12, folic acid, vitamin D, vitamin A, and others. Whether these nutritional difficulties are part of the disease process or are secondary manifestations is not clear.

Neoplastic changes are different: in ulcerative colitis carcinoma develops in the area of inflammation, while in Crohn's the malignancy tends to develop in areas of the bowel where the disease is not clinically active (Lightdale and Sherlock, 1988).

PHARMACEUTICAL TREATMENT

Medical therapy usually has to be directed toward nutritional support. Sulfasalazine and prednisone in combination are less effective than prednisone alone. Unfortunately, many patients treated with steroids cannot have these withdrawn without a flare-up of disease activity. "No drug has been exclusively proven to be useful in prevention of subsequent disease exacerbation" (p. 471). Kirsner (1980) felt that "clinical improvement does seem attributable more to the individual capacity to contain the disease than to any specific drug therapy" (p. xvii). Pharmaceutical therapy is otherwise much the same in ulcerative colitis and in Crohn's disease.

Metronidazole (Flagyl) might be included as a pharmaceutical preparation, but I have chosen to list it, equally appropriately, as an immunosuppressive medication.

IMMUNOSUPPRESSIVE MEDICATION

The results with immunosuppressive therapy seem to be much the same in Crohn's disease as they are in ulcerative colitis. I have already reported Winkelman and Brown's (1965) use of nitrogen mustard in the treatment of ulcerative colitis and Crohn's disease. In 1969, Brooke, Hoffman, and Swarbuck used azathioprine and reported dramatic results with six cases of Crohn's. In 1970, Brooke, Javett, and Davison expanded their work and noted the closures of fistulae in their patients. In 1980, Present, Korelitz, Wisch, Glass, Sachar, and Pasternack conducted a two-year double blind study on 83 chronic cases of Crohn's disease comparing 6-Mercaptopurine with a placebo. Improvement was noted in 67 percent of the drug-treated patients and in 8 percent of those individuals who received the placebo. The drug was more effective than the placebo in closing fistulae. Adverse side effects were present in 10 percent of the patients on the drug.

In 1984, Allison and Pounder reported the use of cyclosporin in Crohn's disease. Methotrexate (Patterson, Ball, and Witske, 1988) has been used with some success in the treatment of inflammatory bowel disease. Present (1989) presented a complete review of the favorable literature on immunosuppressive drugs, and as I have noted, Present et al. (1989) reviewed the side effects and complications in using 6-Mercaptopurine in the treatment of inflammatory bowel disease.

Not all of the literature has been so favorable. Summers, Switz, and Sessions (1979) reported on the National Cooperative Crohn's Disease Study. This study of 569 patients compared prednisone, sulfasalazine, azathioprine, and placebo. Patients on azathioprine showed no statistically significant improvement when compared to placebo. There have been other critical clinical and double-blind studies of immunosuppressive drugs, just as there have been other studies suggesting remarkable short-term improvement. Evidently the closure of fistulae in some cases of Crohn's has been impressive.

There has been some recent interest in the use of metronidazole (Flagyl) in the treatment of Crohn's. Babb (1988b) concluded in an editorial that the efficacy of metronidazole in the treatment of Crohn's disease remains unproved. While he felt that it could help heal perineal disease, which can accompany Crohn's, the side effects of neuropathy, carcinogenicity, and emergence of resistant organisms when metronidazole is taken for long periods of time should indicate that caution be exerted in considering its use.

The future possibilities for the use of immunosuppressive drugs in Crohn's disease are at this point essentially the same as those discussed in our brief review of ulcerative colitis. The complications seem formidable, even though Present et al. (1989) claim that most are reversible or avoidable—at least with 6-Mercaptopurine. Most authors, even the most enthusiastic, feel that these drugs should only be used in chronic disease that has not been responsive to steroids. Long-term and drug-free remissions have not been studied.

A last reflection on immunosuppressive drugs: As one reviews the literature it is apparent that the majority of patients treated with immunosuppressive medications are also continued on steroids and/or sulfasalazine. Thus, one is dealing not only with the complications imposed by the immunosuppressants, but also all of the complications seen in steroid-treated patients.

Surgery

There seem to be greater difficulties in surgical intervention with Crohn's than one finds in surgical treatment of ulcerative colitis. As a matter of fact, at times the complications are monstrous. Frequently recurrent regional enteritis follows surgery. Patients with Crohn's disease are prone to fistulae formation around the areas of surgical intervention.

Surgeons recognize that the surgical treatment of Crohn's disease presents some special problems of its own. An interesting discussion of the difficulties and controversy associated with surgery for Crohn's disease was contained in the correspondence in the journal *Gastroenterology* (1977, pp. 775–779), in response to a paper by Fawaz, Glotzer, Goldman, Dickersin, Gross, and Patterson (1976). The authors felt that the results of colectomy and ileostomy with Crohn's disease were not too unfavorable when compared to similar surgery with ulcerative colitis, and acknowledged that patients with Crohn's disease of the colon required ileostomy revisions more often than did operated patients with ulcerative colitis. They also noted that their diagnostic criteria involved multifactorial analysis—not just histopathological reports.

However, Korelitz (1977) replied that in his experience, 46 percent of 31 cases had recurrent regional ileitis after ileostomy and colectomy performed for Crohn's ileocolitis. He acknowledged different criteria for diagnosis. Sacher, Greenstein, and

Janowitz (1977) felt that Fawaz et al. chose to minimize the differences and they did not recommend proctocolectomy as the primary operation when lesser procedures were available.

In their response, Fawaz, Glotzer, Goldman, Dickersin, and Patterson (1977) disagreed with Korelitz and the other authors, but did observe: "We all must face the fact that there is, at present, no really satisfactory therapy, medical or surgical for CDC [Crohn's] or for that matter UC [ulcerative colitis]" (1977, p. 778).

Korelitz (1979) remarked that "we know also that, following any type of surgery for Crohn's disease, there is a recurrence rate of about 15% per year" (p. 12).

The complicated surgical reconstructions recently developed to follow colectomy in ulcerative colitis are not usually tried with Crohn's disease, which is understandable when one observes the surgical complications described above.

While the topic of surgery of the small intestine is not connected directly with our study of treatment of disease of the colon, it is of interest to mention that because of the tendency of patients with Crohn's to develop neoplastic changes in otherwise apparently healthy gut, and particularly in intestinal segments which have been bypassed, it is frequently recommended that surgery not involve bypassing intestinal segments, and that removal is usually preferable.

All in all, surgery is not as simple a solution to Crohn's disease of the colon as it seems to be in ulcerative colitis. But in either case it is a less than satisfactory solution and does not allow the patient an uncomplicated pattern of life. As I have noted, with Crohn's disease repeated surgery is not uncommon and can be devastating.

While conducting a hospital seminar I visited one young woman who had been through six surgical procedures and whose nutritional requirements were supported only with intravenous feeding. It seemed probable that this would be the only way of maintaining her nutritional needs for the rest of her life.

She suffered from a condition known as "short gut" which often requires total parenteral nutrition. Such a condition can exist when too large a segment, or too many segments of the small intestine have been removed.

Generally, like ulcerative colitis, Crohn's disease is less severe in older patients. Fortunately, unlike ulcerative colitis, it is rare in the childhood years.

Chapter 3
Epidemiology and Genetics of Inflammatory Bowel Disease

EPIDEMIOLOGY

Before the reader's attention is focused on the psychopathological processes that are one dimension of this syndrome's response to the environment, we will discuss a little of what is known about the worldwide distribution of cases of inflammatory processes in the bowel.

As is so often the case, we may learn more by noting the changing patterns of incidence geographically over the last half-century than by pursuing absolute figures, the accuracy of which varies from country to country. However, it is apparent that we are dealing with illnesses developing from rather complex etiological forces.

Măratka (1986) notes that the "incidence of IBD [inflammatory bowel disease] is low in developing countries; . . . that there is little or no evidence of contagion being implicated in the development of IBD; . . . the frequency of IBD has been increasing progressively in recent years; the more rapid increase in western and northern Europe . . . no firm association with any *dietary habit* or *pattern* has been established" (p. 31).

Langman and Logan (1988) agree: "There is good reason for believing that Crohn's disease and ulcerative colitis are common in North America and Northern Europe, in Australia and in white South African populations and colitis and Crohn's disease are probably less common in Southern and Eastern Europe, tropical Asia and Japan, and in China and, probably, in South America, but coherent sets of data tend to be lacking" (p. 165).

While Langman and Logan note that the incidence of both illnesses is less common in Japan and Asia, and along with Mǎratka observe the increasing incidence in western Europe, we should also note the rapidly increasing incidence in some developed Asiatic nations. Admittedly the overall incidence is still a fraction of the incidence in Europe and the United States but changes seem to accrue. Japan, which in the past had relatively few cases of inflammatory bowel disease, has shown a progressive increase in idiopathic proctocolitis between 1965 and 1975 when it began to level off—at least until 1982 (Utsunomiya, Shinohara, Kitahora, Suzuki, and Yokota, 1982, p. 189). The incidence of Crohn's disease also increased quite regularly over the 14 years between 1966 and 1980, but here too, the incidence was still lower than in Europe (Kimura and Sasagawa, 1984, p. 191). It is interesting that the progression in both cases was at a much greater rate in urban population centers than in rural areas.

In Israel there was a marked increase in both illnesses between 1970 and 1980 (Gilat, 1987, p. 239).

When we turn to northern Europe, in Denmark, Sweden, Norway, and the Faeroe Islands both illnesses had parallel increases every year and the increases were far greater in urban areas (Binder, 1957, p. 237).

In the Netherlands (Shivananda, Hordijk, Peña, Ruitenberg, and Mayberry, 1987, p. 245) the situation was much the same with increases and incidence much greater in urban areas than in the countryside.

Statistics for the rest of northern Europe roughly replicate those noted above.

Mendelhoff and Calkins (1988, pp. 3–34) report that women are at increased risk over men for inflammatory bowel disease. However, Langman and Logan (1988, p. 166) note that if there are differences overall in disease frequency between men and women these are likely to be small. In general children under ten years of age are unlikely to develop Crohn's disease, but ulcerative colitis is not infrequent. From 10 to 20 years of age the incidence of ulcerative colitis outpaces that of Crohn's, but the incidence of the latter illness progresses year by year during this decade. According to these two authors, from the ages of 20 to 50 the two diseases are almost identical in annual incidence. Others observe that Crohn's is rare after 40.

Mendelhoff and Calkins (1988) either contradict or update Goodman and Sparberg's figures. The latter noted (1978, p. 7) that the annual incidence of Crohn's disease in northern Europe is 3 to 5 per 100,000 population as opposed to ulcerative colitis which is 5 to 10 per 100,000 population. The incidence of ulcerative colitis had been relatively stable since the 1950s while the incidence of Crohn's has been "rising by two or three-fold between 1955 and 1973."

Bayless (1979) observed the host characteristics in Crohn's disease and noted that the average age of the patients was 27 (p. 21), that 10 percent had the illness before age 15, and that it was unusual to develop the illness after 40 (p. 22).

GENETIC POSSIBILITIES

Purrmann (1987) has summarized some of the basic research and observations.

> Our current knowledge of IBD suggests that genetic and environmental factors interact. Data on recurrence in first degree relatives of patients with IBD exclude an autosomal dominant (50% risk in siblings) or an autosomal recessive (25% risk in siblings) inheritance. An autosomal recessive inheritance with low penetrance is also extremely improbable. Sex-linked transmission is excluded by the fact that IBD is roughly as common in men as in women. The hypothesis of a polygenic inheritance with threshold effect fits the epidemiological data best . . . Only if a critical number of predisposing genes is exceeded and certain environmental factors interact does IBD become manifest [pp. 209–210].

Kidd and Morton (1989) point out that psychosomatic disorders, in general, are not determined by genetic factors alone . . . these disorders are complex . . . although this is an area of genetic research that has witnessed great progress, it still 'has a long way to go' " (p. 385). "When a trait has been shown to be complex, i.e., when both genetic and nongenetic factors are known to contribute to etiology and pathogenesis, many simple methods for the identification of etiological factors are no longer appropriate" (p. 388). "Nature-nurture arguments are not the issue. Rather the question is which specific inherited factors interact with which nongenetic factors to result in the phenotype, i.e., the observable trait or disorder?" (p. 386).

Because inflammatory bowel disease presents no specific characteristics linked directly to a specific genetic pattern (as in Huntington's chorea or Tay-Sach's disease) the interaction of a polygenic background with environmental factors is intriguing. When we realize that we are investigating complex pathological conditions from two parallel platforms of observation: the psyche (mind) and the physical (physiology including cerebral states [see chapters 6 and 7]). We can foresee both further complications and greater clarity.

Koranyi (1989) had some feeling for the possible confusion when he wrote:

> What is referred to as "genetic predisposition," which determines individual responses to "stress resistance," is a hazy concept which, as such may not even exist on gene levels. . . . In general terms the notion of genetic disposition remains an enigma. This, of course, does not mean that physiological responses are not genetically controlled. Quite the contrary, but there are a multitude of responses controlled polygenetically, the abstract and non biological collection of which is referred to as "genetic disposition" [pp. 268–269].

Our interest in the psychiatric field of observation directs our attention to the subjective world of the patient where we formulate psychic experience in traditional psychoanalytic terms, which are often reduced to such abstractions as drives and defenses.

Freud (1937) and Schur (1955) are among the countless psychoanalytic explorers who have commented on the importance of heredity, disposition, and the probability of differences in the strengths of the aggressive and libidinal impulses between one individual and another (the psychological "genetic predisposition"). There is the strong probability that individual differences in the utilization of defense may be traced to genetic endowments as well as to environmental factors.

The vicissitudes in environmental evolution of genetic or constitutional endowments are highly significant in our studies of patients with inflammatory bowel disease. It has been repeatedly demonstrated (Murray, 1930a,b; Daniels, 1941, 1942; M. Sperling, 1946, 1978b; Engel, 1955; Savitt, 1977; Hogan, 1989, to name only a few) that patients with inflammatory disease of the colon suffer from unusually intense conflicts involving aggressive impulses (drives) with sadistic fantasies. The unfortunate assumption that either the predisposition to intense aggression and corresponding defensive adaptation is inherited, or that intrapsychic is only an ubiquitous result of conflict within the family environment, would seem to be a false opposition of abstract alternatives.

A correct reading of our data should give us an indication of the balance between the oversimplified "nature" and "nurture."

Freud (1937), in accordance with his many previous assertions of the importance of genetic contributions to the neuroses, emphasized (pp. 240–241) that the more pathological the genetic endowment, the less the environmental traumatization necessary to produce a neurosis. This general observation can, of course, be applied to somatic responses. Any predisposition to neurotic conflict or somatization of conflicts does not rule out the possibility of an accompanying specific predisposition to intestinal responses of an inflammatory nature.

As Schur (1955), discussing psychosomatic responses in general (and dermatological responses specifically), noted:

The more a certain way of organ response is genetically determined, the less is the relative importance of the neurosis. The relative importance of genetically determined organ response differs not only with different entities but may show considerable variation within the same entity. . . . The genetic factor . . . will determine the *type* of response, yet in the entire constellation the emphasis will be on the neurotic conflict [pp. 157–158].

Investigators may discover that a pattern of susceptibility to somatic responses in general may be determined by a genetic predisposition (Schur, 1955; Wilson, Hogan, and Mintz, 1983; Wilson and Mintz, 1989).

Whatever the specifics, the neurological apparatus and the psychological apparatus appear to evolve and mature in a parallel fashion along somewhat predestined (genetic or constitutional) patterns molded by environmental forces.

While psychoanalysts will continue to focus attention on the vicissitudes of psychic structures, physiological geneticists will undoubtedly train their sights on correlates between chromosomes and physiological artifacts.

Probably the greatest errors in any clinical investigation arise from our rush to judgment in detailing a single etiological factor or agent. We are not dealing with nature or nurture, but with the complex relationship between the two as seen from various spheres of observation.

Chapter 4
What Is Not Idiopathic Inflammatory Disease of the Colon

There are many pathological conditions of the colon and intestines, some of which present interesting problems in differential diagnoses of ulcerative colitis and Crohn's disease, but which usually are totally unrelated.

Vascular disease and anomalies are not infrequent (Bynum and Jacobson, 1988). Within this group the one condition that might concern us in differential diagnosis is eschemic colitis, which can result from arterial occlusion, cardiac pathology, shock, dehydration, and so on (Norris, 1977).

I once observed a single incidence of "Crohn's ileitis" in a middle-aged man that I suspected was an ischemic segment of intestine resulting from arterial occlusion. Following surgery there were no related complications, nor have there been any recurrences. More important, the patient's subjective psychological makeup was not of a type that commonly accompanies Crohn's disease.

Eisenberg, Montgomery, and Margulis (1979) had some interesting comments about presumed inflammatory bowel disease in the elderly: "We propose that . . . in older patients with no history of bowel disease, colitis pathologically diagnosed as ulcerative or granulomatous colitis actually represents various stages of ischemic colitis" (p. 1113) and conclude: "In these patients, the clinical presentation and subsequent course are

35

the only basis for a diagnosis that cannot otherwise be proved" (p. 1117).

There are other conditions (Jewell, 1988, pp. 549–556; Thayer and DeNucci, 1988) of a more general nature that may involve the colon in various ways. Neurological diseases such as Parkinsonism and multiple sclerosis can give rise to symptoms in the gut. Hypothyroidism; hyperthyroidism; Addison's disease; systemic lupus erythematosis; polyarteritis nodosa; diabetes; hemodialysis or kidney transplant with colon ulcers; leukemia; and sickle cell disease are all possible sources of colon pathology.

Amyloidosis; pelvic endometriosis; collagenous colitis; cathartic colon following extensive use of laxatives, including melanosis coli; anemia; induced intestinal lesions; radiation colitis; drug-induced colitis; or nonspecific ulcers of the colon, rectum, and anus can each occasionally present diagnostic problems. Infections with either bacteria or parasites obviously often present acute or chronic inflammatory symptoms (Quinn and Schuffler, 1988, pp. 439–481; Zaiman, Frierson, and Shorter, 1988, pp. 403–506). Among the bacterial infections one might find are shigella, salmonella, complyobactor (vibrio fetus), various strains of escheria coli, vibrio parahaemolyticus, staphlococcus, clostridium perfringens, clostridium difficile in antibiotic-associated pseudomembranous enterocolitis, chlamydia trachomatis, syphilis, nisseria gonorrhea, mycobacterium tuberculosis.

Parasitic infections may include nematodes: tricharis trichiuri (whipworm), enterobius vermicularis (pinworm), strongyloidiasis stercoralis (thread worm), and schistosomiasis. The protozoal possibilities may include one of the various strains of amebiasis, dianthro ameba fragilis, and acute or chronic Chagas disease.

Venereal infections, some of which have already been listed, may be present, most commonly in homosexual men. Women, too, may involve the anus in sexual activity, and there is always the questionable possibility of disease transmission from the vagina over the perineal area to the anus.

The physician has to face the question of idiopathic inflammatory bowel disease complicated by a coexisting bacterial or parasitic infection.

One important disease entity presenting a problem of differential diagnosis is the acute stage of diverticulitis (Schwartz and Graham, 1988, pp. 519–536). Diverticulitis has occasionally been seen in combination with ulcerative colitis.

The not uncommon irritable colon may be associated with frequent stools, nonbloody diarrhea, or mucous colitis. This condition is not of immediate interest despite its observable simultaneous emotional concomitants and precursors. In medical literature irritable colon or what is often known as mucous colitis are ordinarily totally separated as entities from inflammatory disease of the colon.

The usual case of irritable colon is just that, whether transient or chronic. However, I have observed that some psychoanalytic patients who develop inflammatory bowel disease give a history of what could be called irritable colon in childhood or early adolescence. Again, there are further difficulties in definition and evaluation because patients successfully treated with psychoanalytic psychotherapy for inflammatory bowel disease often develop transient symptoms similar to those of irritable colon as they give up their ulcerative colitis. It is probable in such patients under treatment that one is dealing with incidental colonic activity, not with a disease entity, "irritable colon."

There are probably some other illnesses that can feign the symptoms of idiopathic inflammatory disease of the colon. Usually ulcerative colitis, ulcerative proctitis, and Crohn's disease involving the distal colon are not difficult diagnostic problems. However, Crohn's ileitis or ileocolitis may present some difficulty. When bleeding and diarrhea are not present, a more exhaustive investigation is necessary.

Chapter 5
Physiological and Psychopathological Considerations

INTRODUCTION

Physicians have shown diverse attitudes toward the existence of psychopathology or its role as an accompanying variable in inflammatory diseases of the colon. Some ignore totally the observations and treatment results of psychiatric and psychoanalytic investigators. Banks, Present, and Steiner (1983), among others, deny any emotional conflicts as concomitants in the inflammatory reaction patterns of these illnesses. Unfortunately, their conclusions clearly represent the position of the National Foundation of Ileitis and Colitis in its *Crohn's Disease and Ulcerative Colitis Fact Book,* a publication directed at a lay audience.

When I use the concept of emotional concomitants here I am referring to what has commonly been viewed as emotional etiology, I am not referring to incidental or "resulting" (somatopsychic in interactionist language)[1] reactions. Emotional conflict

---

[1]Interactionism describes a particular relationship between mind and body, as though mind (subjective data) were an entity—as opposed to a particular collection of data—and body (physical, neurophysiological data) seen as another entity—and not another particular collection of data. Interactionism describes interaction between two entities—mind and body—and implies the independence of each; although with linguistic cant or metaphor, identity is sometimes claimed within the interactionist concept. Often causality is an important element of interactionism: mind causes physical activity or brain causes mind (mind is a function of brain). What is seldom acknowl-

is no more solely the result of physical distress than is physical symptomatology solely the result of emotional conflict. We are observing paralled data from parallel fields of observations.

Despite the disclaimers of some observers a substantial number of investigators do recognize the important relationship between emotional conflict and inflammatory disease of the colon. If we return to the commonly utilized therapeutic activities of physicians who treat these illnesses, the literature seems to indicate that the majority are in favor of supportive psychotherapy as an ancillary help. Some recommend continuous supportive psychotherapy. Some in each group specifically warn against the use of psychoanalysis or psychoanalytic psychotherapy. Very few recommend either approach as a primary therapeutic modality despite favorable results from numerous investigators (see chapter 12).

Studies of the psychopathology of inflammatory disease of the colon seem to be endless in number and unlimited in variety. Our interest is not in the myriad investigations of biochemical or physiological details that may or may not relate to that cerebral cortical-hypothalamic-adrenocortical system which might parallel the subjective psychodynamic systems accompanying the pathophysiology of inflammatory disease of the colon.

The attempts at quantification and objectification of psychiatric diagnoses, psychological profiles, psychological evaluations, and psychological tests of these patients are uncountable, and, for the most part, of little concern to us.

In my attempt to present a few important early psychophysiological studies and very few representational examples of psychiatric and psychological opinions, I begin by mentioning an early investigator, George Daniels (1941, 1942, 1944; Karush and Daniels, 1953; Daniels, O'Connor, Karush, Moses, Flood, and Lepore, 1962; Karush, Daniels, O'Connor, and Stern,

---

edged is that causality denotes a temporal sequence, and with interactionism one is by definition infering a temporal relationship between body and mind. Further discussion of the concept is found in chapters 6 and 7.

1968, 1969) who made enormous contributions to our understanding of the diseases of the large gut; all summarized in the monograph *Psychotherapy in Chronic Ulcerative Colitis* (Karush, Daniels, Flood, and O'Connor, 1977).

The contributions of G. L. Engel to the study of ulcerative colitis are notable (1952, 1954a,b, 1955, 1956, 1958, 1961a,b, 1962, 1967, 1973; Engel and Schmale, 1967). In his early work (1954a) he observed that "the most frequent earliest abnormality was the passage of blood" (p. 497). While ulcerative colitis was generally thought of as a diarrheal disease, he noted that only Sperling among those investigators of psychosomatic hypothesis concerned herself with bleeding as a fundamental characteristic (p. 496).

In the same paper he noted that "chronic constipation, either severe or moderate" was a frequent premorbid, or could be, an initiating symptom (p. 499). "In all [patients with constipation], frequent use of cathartics or enemas, or both, had been considered necessary, having been initiated in childhood by a parent and continued by the patient in adult life" (p. 499), observing that his patients had paid excessive attention to bowel behavior in childhood and were subject to early toilet training. Many displayed rectal spasm and brief episodes of diarrhea (perhaps irritable colon?) as premorbid symptoms.

During the same year (1954b) he reviewed some of the literature associating affective states with colonic activity, but he felt totally blocked on the "jump from the psychic phenomena to the physical phenomena at the end organ" (p. 431). He felt it was "conceptually most difficult" (p. 431).

He later (1955) gave an excellent review of the literature before that date, noting:

> [Ulcerative colitis patients fall into a] population group having predominately pregenital character traits especially compulsive and dependent features; they show a defect in their capacity to relate to people, with a tendency to retain features of their early mother–child symbiotic relation; there is a failure to resolve this symbiotic relationship; which genetically also appears to be related to the distinctive characteristic of one parent, usually

mother who cannot relinquish this relationship with her child; sexual maturity is not achieved . . . ulcerative colitis develops in settings in which the important relationship in fact or fantasy is threatened or actually disrupted, when at the same time the patient feels helpless to cope with the new situations; remissions occur when the affective relationship is again achieved; . . . there is a vulnerability to psychotic reactions greater than the general population . . . [p. 246].

Engel also noted (1956):

[A] high proportion of patients with ulcerative colitis also suffer with headaches. . . . [I]t was found that the headaches occurred when the patients felt in control, had taken an active stand, made a decision, thought something through. . . . In none of these instances did the patients feel helpless or afraid and in none did they feel their important relationships seriously jeopardized. *In all of these examples there was evidence of strong conscious or unconscious aggressive or sadistic impulses.* . . . Bleeding, on the other hand, occurred . . . when the patient was feeling to varying degrees helpless, hopeless, or despairing . . . with the appearance of bleeding, the patient would feel overwhelmed and give up [pp. 334–335; emphasis added].

In spite of his astute observations on the psychopathology of ulcerative colitis patients, Engel seemed to disregard psychoanalysis or psychoanalytic psychotherapy as a treatment of choice and recommended continuous supportive psychotherapy. "The susceptibility to the disease probably persists for the rest of life and until medicine discovers a way to influence the basic biologic defect no real expectation of cure is possible" (1958, p. 333). He adds, "One will do well never to discharge a patient with ulcerative colitis" (p. 335).

In 1958 (p. 336) he restated his position that such patients suffer or anticipate, consciously or unconsciously, the loss of an important love object and that they respond by feeling helpless, hopeless, or despairing which may be accompanied by bleeding.

He seems to have evaluated his patients with a team approach and a statistical point of view. He has given us a beautiful description of the psychological characteristics, object relations, family dynamics, and sexual and marital adjustments of patients with inflammatory disease of the colon, but at the same time he continued to depend on medical treatment, using supportive psychotherapy as an auxiliary tool (1961a, 1962, 1967, 1973).

Engel was trained both as an internist and a psychoanalyst, but it appears he had little faith in the psychoanalytic method for treatment of these patients. Nevertheless, for any psychoanalytic investigator or physician psychoanalyst who treats inflammatory bowel disease, the pioneering work of Engel is of utmost importance from both its psychological and physiological points of view.

Almy is another investigator who has contributed much to our knowledge of the colon under stress (Almy and Tulin, 1947; Almy, Kern, and Tulin, 1949; Almy, Hinkle, Berle, and Kern, 1949; Almy, 1961a,b; Almy and Lewis, 1963; Almy and Sherlock, 1966; Almy, 1975).

In his early work (Almy and Tulin, 1947; Almy, Kern, and Tulin, 1949) Almy and his coworkers utilized normal volunteers, using proctoscopic observation and inlying balloons as the volunteers were placed under stress of cold, pain, and headaches. He discovered spasm of the sigmoid colon, blanching of the mucosa, or hyperemia of the mucosa. He also observed pallor of the skin, hypertension, sweating, sighing, and so on. Some patients showed increased secretions on the mucosae.

He and his colleagues (Almy, Kern, and Tulin, 1949) investigated the production of sigmoid spasm in patients with spastic constipation when under stress. He concluded that "the fundamental abnormality in the patient with spastic constipation lies not in the behavior of his colon but in his susceptibility to stress producing life situations" (p. 449).

His work took him into the area of ulcerative colitis (Almy, 1961a,b), where he utilized kynographic recordings with a single balloon or approximated balloons in normal subjects and 45 individuals with ulcerative colitis (1961a, p. 300).

[Sixty percent of the ulcerative colitis patients had] significantly reduced phasic activity, defined as "straight line" tracing. . . . an additional type of wave . . . 8 to 10 times longer in duration and 2 or 3 times greater in amplitude than the average contraction. . . . [This has never] been observed in a resting tracing of an individual without ulcerative colitis. . . . It has been possible to identify this same phenomenon of suppression of phasic activity . . . transitionally in individuals exposed to disturbing emotionally charged interviews, . . . [and] by the injection of potent cholinergic agents [pp. 299–303].

He further noted:

In no other diarrheal disease have we observed a motility pattern of this type steadily present in the resting colon. . . . [We have] failed to find it in regional ileitis, in sprue, in functional diarrhea, and in the subsiding phases of infectious enteritis, . . . a sort of *posture* of the colon, a continued readiness for defecation [p. 304].

His clinical evaluations (1961b) and his work with Sherlock (Almy and Sherlock, 1966) were of note for their speculations on postnatal influences and possible genetic determinants.

Almy's 1975 paper is important for many reasons, but his definition of "psychosomatic" is of particular interest:

The term psychosomatic is here used to describe any reaction of the organism to environmental stress in which objective bodily changes and emotional disturbances occur in *parallel*. . . . This concept implies a biological response of the organism as a whole, an arousal of its general defensive reaction patterns, even though it may appear to be concentrated in the function of a single organ, such as the colon. It *denies that the emotions themselves cause the bodily change* . . . they are merely the affective features of the total reaction [pp. 37–38; emphasis added; see chapters 6 and 7].

Almy, like Engel, recommended supportive psychotherapy with medical management, anxiety reducing drugs, antidepressants and sedatives. He felt:

Analytic methods make far greater demands on the patient and at some point require the therapist to become an unsympathetic or even threatening figure, to enable the patient to work through a long repressed emotional conflict. Such a relationship is often counter productive in the patient with active disease and may be associated with a clear-cut exacerbation of symptoms [p. 44].

Despite Almy's feelings about prognosis and treatment, which do not completely agree with ours, he has contributed a prodigious amount of informative and imaginative work in the study of inflammatory disease of the colon.

One study by Fullerton, Kollar, and Caldwell (1962) attempted statistical studies with arbitrary categories of arbitrary measurements. "The authors reject hypotheses which focus on particular aspects of the pan psychopathology in order to establish symbolic meaning for the somatic pathology or to link the illness to specific difficulties in the mother child relationship during a circumscribed phase of development" (p. 463). One could also make the observation that any study arbitrarily eliminating the important contributions of other authors starts with an admitted bias.

Clifford Hawkins (1983) voiced an opinion often found in the literature. "A psychosomatic cause is assumed rather than proved, and the current view is that psychological factors, though important, are not the cause" (p. 445).

Bayless (1979) repeated the familiar theme. "I do not believe that such factors are primary. I think that stress obviously has been involved in some flare-ups in some patients but there does not seem to be any primary personality disorder" (p. 22).

Some authors, like Lennard-Jones in his etiology of nonspecific inflammatory bowel disease (1981), do not even mention observations of emotional factors either as presumed "*causal*" or as simultaneous concomitants of the physical activity.

Roth (1976) felt that "formal psychotherapy may be necessary for the seriously disturbed patient with severe obsessive-compulsive states, depression, schizophrenic or paranoid reactions, or suicidal attempts. However, psychoanalytic methods to explore the psychodynamics may be dangerous during the acute phase of ulcerative colitis" (p. 714). Like many others holding this view he is by implication acknowledging the existence of exceedingly important subjective conflicts concomitant to the physical symptoms. He also acknowledges a profound effect of psychoanalysis on the physical symptoms.

One could continue ad infinitum with absences, qualified acknowledgments, or cautionary tales about the psychological treatment of inflammatory bowel disease. However, occasionally one runs across diverting, if tangential, clinical papers.

Stephen Eisenhammer (1982) commented on a nine-year follow-up of "A case of acute fulminating colitis" with failure of chemotherapeutic treatment. Electroconvulsive therapy instead of proctocolectomy was decided upon. The patient responded well and the reason for choice of treatment is fully argued. The author was led to believe that "this condition as well as associated ones can only arise in a person with a slight congenital aberration in his thalamo-hypothalamic region. It is also postulated that this simple small defect is 'reversible' and [can be] completely eliminated and corrected by this shock therapy resulting in a permanent cure" (p. 10). One could only wish that our comprehension of this disease were so complete and understandable from a neurological, psychological, and general physiological view point. When an observer is committed to what one might call a mechanical point of view and will with one case reduce an explanation to an overly simplified, undocumentable neurophysiological explanation, ignoring every other frame of observation or organization of explanation, one cannot put much faith in it. It is of interest that this patient recovered with a form of treatment commonly used for psychiatric illness. I would not use this case as a recommendation for electroshock therapy in colitis—or, as a matter of fact, for any other condition.

I trust the reader will recognize that I don't take Bucaille's suggestions very seriously when I quote from his paper, "Selective Frontal Surgery in Digestive Pathology" (1964): "hemorragic recto colitis is a major indication of this type of operation"

(p. 229). The surgery that he recommends is "electrocoagulation of the supero-internal portion of the frontal white matter . . . interrupt[ing] certain association routes between the frontal cortical region and the thalamo-hypothalamic regions which control the neuro-autonomic nervous system" (p. 229). We can see that although very destructive, it is a simple, dramatic approach to an extremely complex problem.

In an entirely different clinical direction we might look at the psychopathology of the siamang gibbon. Stout and Snyder (1969) wrote an article on four deceased animals of this species from two different zoos. "According to 'zoo lore' a siamang gibbon will frequently 'pine away' and die following the loss of a long time cage mate." Animals who died with chronic debilitation under these conditions in two separate locations were autopsied and lesions identical to those of human ulcerative colitis were discovered. They were cultured for shigella, salmonella, and pathogenic coliform bacteria, but none were found.

We can hypothesize that at least one other species can react to the loss of a love object or its equivalent with a fatal inflammatory disease of the colon. I am not being totally facetious when I claim that I make no pretense of having come to any conclusion about subjective symbolism in siamang gibbons. There may be organic changes of a psychosomatic nature without clearly traceable accompanying symbolization (Sperling, 1952; Sarnoff, 1989).

On the other hand, symbolization is only one aspect of subjective thought (the activities of the mind). Inasmuch as the siamang has no access to speech, we are unable to make any judgment about the subjective thought processes that may parallel the neurophysiological or physiological activities of the siamang gibbon.

This small sample of the many observations from a number of clinical investigators gives a representative sample of conclusions drawn by nonpsychoanalytic observers. Chapter 12 introduces clinical studies from psychoanalytically oriented physicians.

Part II
Psychosomatic Considerations

Chapter 6
Introduction to Psyche and Soma

Man has struggled with the mind–body problem throughout most of recorded history. I hope that I am not being presumptuous in calling attention to certain discoveries relating to this problem in the realms of physiology and psychology. Some have made notable contributions to our understanding of the dimensions of investigative efforts in these fields (Feigl, 1950, 1958; Graham, 1967). Their work allows the thoughtful empiricist to recognize that solutions to the problem are available if one carefully examines one's sources of data (see chapter 7) and one's linguistics as scrupulously as one examines the data itself. Since it is of such importance to our studies of the psychology of the colitis patient as well as to the entire field of psychosomatics, I shall devote Part II to some general and specific discussion of psyche and soma.

In even the most important contributions to the field of the neurosciences there is often a feeling of perplexity about psychology and its place in or alongside the field of neurophysiology. Our confusion is sometimes acknowledged, but the basis for it is more usually ignored or denied, and the resultant difficulties in handling the data are overlooked.

There have been numerous attempts to explain away the problem. The term *psychosomatic medicine* has been inappropriately broadened to include such labels as biopsychosocial in an effort to obliterate some of the contradictions attributed to the term *psychosomatic*. Some investigators have been attracted to

51

the speculations of the psychologist von Bertalanffy, and his systems theory, in an attempt to find a place for what they regard as an errant science. In the same and different contexts terms such as *regulation* and *disregulation* have had their usually limited meanings modified and elaborated into explanatory theoretical positions.

The basis for all of this head-scratching lies in an agreed-upon observation—the duality of our sources of data. Due to a devotion to false parsimony, few physicians or others have been willing to admit that the duality of their sources of data is real.

It is at this point that I wish to offer a contribution to an understanding of the mind–body enigma, the way to which has been paved by the proponents of parallelism, who used "isomorphism" as a verbal bridge and explanation of the apparent contradictions in the mind–body problem. Feigl (1950, 1958) proposed an alternative dual language postulate and Graham (1967) proposed "linguistic parallelism." Feigl and Graham both saw the duality and the parallel nature of the language used for the correct communication of data and its organized derivatives.

It is clear that we are dealing with data witnessed and/or recorded from two different observational viewpoints: (1) data experienced by the subjective self (mind); and (2) data perceived by outside observation, in this case, the soma including our observations of the body and brain.

In the case of (1) mind, the data from the subjective self, we include any number of subclassifications: emotional, religious, psychological, etc. The data may lend itself to organization, abstraction, theoretical formulation, interpretation, etc., and still remain in that category—mind.

If we turn to the (2) body we include all of the innumerable physical and physiological subclassifications. We must note here that in this objective world of interest we include the data from the panorama of outside observations whether it relates to brain, to body, to elephants, or to chemistry. Here too, organization, abstractions, theoretical formulations, and so on, are all part of the objective physical (in its broadest sense) world. It makes no difference whether our "objective" observations are personal or through instrumentation: the data is derived from observation of the world outside of our subjective selves.

Although Feigl and Graham have brilliantly led the way to an understanding and explanation of the parallel position of linguistics in recognition of the parallel position of mind and body, I intend to contribute my own observations on the two parallel sources of data implicit in the words "mind" and "body." I will demonstrate that, although we conceive of "mind" and "body" as irreducible entities, they are words used to describe an accumulation of data that we take for granted.

To repeat: In our observations of nature and life our data is derived from two (dual) fields of observation: (1) the subjective (mind) and (2) the external world (body, brain and whatever). In such observations we can demonstrate parallel fields of observation (sources of information), i.e., mind and brain (psyche and physical). The parallel data that we obtain may be simultaneous and/or synchronous, i.e., (1) the sensation of fear with palpitations may be simultaneous with our (2) physiological studies of tachycardia.

Much of the confusion may lie in our perception of, and insistence on, the body (brain) and mind as entities or series of entities. While in popular parlance and by common definition they are entities, what is neglected is the semantic recognition that any entity, however named, is a noun and a recognition of a high order of abstraction that has evolved over unknown time. The "entity" is an accumulation of data endlessly modified over an indefinite period. We are inclined to toss such nouns around as though they were irreducible and timeless.

For the most part traditional thinking has thrown all diverse data (those "entities" as commonly perceived) into a sequential line of presentation and causality, i.e., "fear can in some instances cause tachycardia," in which the demonstrable duality and parallelism is obscured.

Among the many reasons for the investigators' need to avoid any recognition of the dual and parallel sources of data is the intuitive recognition that there is a single process involved (Deutsch, 1922, p. 139; Cobb, 1963, pp. 138–139). Various proponents who intuitively sense an identity have handled their legitimate wishes for parsimony in various ways. In most cases the duality of two coordinate observable data bases and the parallel nature of the linguistic communication is ignored or denied by linguistic structure and metaphor. In chapter 7, I show how Stanley Cobb utilized causality (the linguistic construction, "function of") as an ostensible salute to parsimony. He failed to recognize the parallel positions of his data bases. Fortunately, it is demonstrable that such an identity can be designated (or abstracted) by the recognition that in psychosomatic considerations one is examining parallel sets of simultaneous data.

Felix Deutsch (1922) provides an example of an intuitive recognition of the identity of the psychological self and the physiological apparatus. But he denies the possibility of parallelism and does not recognize that simultaneous parallel data can represent an identity. Deutsch's protests are in some way understandable. As long as one sees parallel data (sources of data) as parallel entities it is impossible to conceive of an identity of dual entities, even if parallel. Fortunately, such an identity can be implied if one recognizes that one is witnessing parallel and simultaneous sets of data.

In many instances the identity is self-evident, and the parallel nature of the observations is ignored. Some investigators acknowledge the parallel nature of the observations with a certain puzzlement (Almy, 1975). Others recognize the identity, and in order to maintain a parsimonious feeling about the situation deny the parallel nature of their observations (Deutsch, 1922). When the data are simultaneous and parallel (i.e., subjective pain, when it accompanies observed afferent neural discharge from stimulated skin receptors and resulting cerebral activity), we assume an identity of process. In this illustration the data, described as felt subjective pain, are simultaneous and parallel to the data observed and described as receptor stimulation, the afferent neuronal impulse, and the cerebral integration. We may presume an identity of process or event with descriptions of the psychic and physical coordinates. The sources of our data are parallel and dual. There is no temporal (causal) sequence between the two sources of data.

This duality is not just apparent. It is real and it represents different platforms of observation. Each observational viewpoint has its own language: the word *pain*, representing the subjective experience, is parallel with the terms *pain receptor stimulation, nerve impulse,* and *cerebral integration,* representing observed physical activity. I also intend to demonstrate that not only can this be, but that recognizing the parallel observations will give us a greater appreciation and better understanding of, and more uses for the data.

Even the psychologist von Bertalanffy acknowledged such a duality when he was willing to (1964) "postulate an *isomorphism* between the constructs of psychology and neurophysiology" (p. 41; emphasis added).

Isomorphism, incidentally, is a descriptive explanatory term utilized in many sciences such as biology, mathematics, and crystallography. It usually represents an event that can exist in two parallel and sometimes reflected forms. It has become the traditional explanation for identity in traditional psychophysiological parallelism. It may be looked upon as the concept that the entity "mind" reflects (is identical to?) the entity "brain." The concept of isomorphism is an awkward one. On the one hand it acknowledges the identity of mind and brain and acknowledges the parallel data observable in that identity. Yet it treats mind and brain as though they were two separate objects, and explains the identity as though these "entities" reflected one another. Feigl (1958) attempted to explain and dispense with the construct isomorphism in his criticism of traditional psychophysiological parallelism, and Feigl proceeded to recognize parallel languages rather than parallel entities or processes. Von Bertalanffy (1964, 1968) used isomorphism as a convenient word to explain away the duality and traditional parallelistic position of the mind–body problem. He then ignored this conundrum and proceeded to place man in an abstract spatial relationship between his physiology, on the one hand, and out-side environmental phenomena on the other.

The specific duality between the subjective and the external world is empirically evident, but it is a duality of the sources of data (traditional entities). It has little to do with "Cartesian dualism," as von Bertalanffy described it. Cartesian dualism is a carefully defined form of primitive *interactionism*. It claims that mind causes and/or influences body, and that body causes and/or influences mind. It is in direct opposition to any paral-lelistic doctrine. Suffice it to say that Descartes' "thinking sub-stance" (1637, p. 127; 1644, pp. 201, 210) and "extended sub-stance" (1644, pp. 208, 210) are of historical importance only in that he proposed, described, and explained a specific duality of entities, entities which were postulated to be separate and even in opposition to each other. He implied a causal (temporal) relationship between his "thinking" and "extended" substances, reflected today in the doctrine of *independence* and in the doc-trine of *interactionism*. The mind–body problem existed then as it may appear to now, and has been explored and interpreted by philosophers before and after Descartes.

One hopes that recognition of the duality in the sources of data may relieve us of the forced assumption of the usual medi-cal (and Cartesian) idea of dual interacting entities. We may even find that we can conceive of an identity for mind and nervous system while still recognizing the duality in the sources and description of our data.

In the field of philosophy, psychophysiological parallelism with isomorphism has long been offered as a method of under-standing the mind–body problem, but as long as the psyche and soma were seen as concrete entities the idea of parallelism was usually ignored or rejected in medical, psychological, and physiological circles. Parallelism is the recognition that there are parallel avenues of observation of psychic and somatic data. But with original psychoneurophysiological parallelism the em-phasis was on the parallel nature of the events observed, not on the parallel fields of observation.

Felix Deutsch (1922) exemplifies some of this doubt and confusion when describing a subjective sensation preceding a conversion reaction: "Whatever the case may be, the concept of a psychophysical parallelism must be rejected, for nothing parallel occurs here. The temporal coincidence of psychic and physical manifestations develops from the *identity* of these processes" (p. 69). One has to agree totally with this identity of process. On the other hand, one must question Deutsch's concept of psychophysiological parallelism. This example does represent parallelism, whether seen linguistically or with traditional isomorphism. But only with the recognition of parallel data can we recognize such an identity of an event involving mind and body. It is interesting that Deutsch clearly describes the dual sources of his data and rightfully proceeds to declare an identity. In this particular case Deutsch did not indulge in interactionism: the assumption that the psychic caused the physical, which certainly would not allow his justified concept of "identity."

Stanley Cobb (1963), in his attempt to maintain a monistic position, wrote of the mind–body problem, taking the authoritative position that "there is no such problem" (pp. 36, 138–140). He insisted upon remaining above confrontation and conflict.

There are innumerable examples of confusion and self-contradiction by astute and able investigators when they attempted to present their data and thoughts in meaningful contexts. However, most investigators have accepted the interactionist doctrines of mind causing body, body causing mind, or one being the function of the other. In so doing they have accepted a temporal sequence between mind and body.

I hope to help clarify some of the confusion. One is dealing here with the organization of psychosomatic data. In the study of man's relationship with himself and the world, on both a psychological and physical plane, one has to acknowledge the importance of social, behavioristic, epidemiological, and other data bases as one must in understanding any medical entity. I do not believe that widening the definition of psychosomatic to include all of these other observational frames of reference helps us in any way to understand the totally justified, but more limited, idea of psychosomatic investigation. Biopsychosocial is a fine contraction for the study of all of medicine, but biopsychosocial is not synonymous with psychosomatic. I am not even sure that it helps us place man more accurately in life's various categories of internal and environmental abstractions.

Reiser (1975) illustrated the linear interactionist position when he discussed "mechanisms by which the CNS [central nervous system] is able to mediate between higher mental functions (and psychological responses to psychosocial events) on the one hand and the maintenance of metabolic processes and integrity of body tissues on the other" (p. 489). I go no further with Reiser's description of "man existing in a bio-psycho-social field . . ." (p. 492), but try to clarify the interactionist logic behind this linear causal thinking and positioning. With the recognition of linguistic parallelism the use of simultaneous data from the parallel sources mind and body is clear, useful and explainable. There is little use in spending time looking for a neurone that carries emotion, or a chain of neurones that change social perceptions into physiological activity, if we recognize that our physical data encompass only a physical understanding of neurones that transmit physical energy when we are in the neurophysiological areas of observation. These neurones transmit impulses. On the other hand, emotion (mind) is a subjective experience that is *felt* in the area of introspective and/ or psychic observation, and is described in its own languages. It does not travel along neurones. Emotions, as subjective data, may or may not be communicated to an observer for recording, abstracting, or explaining. Transduction in neurones is an attempt to define something that does not exist.

Chapter 7
Psyche and Soma: Linguistics, Causality, and Linguistic Parallelism

Graham (1967) called the mind–body problem "a hoary old philosophical chestnut" (p. 52), and it has presented complicated religious, philosophical, and scientific questions for a variety of partisans over the ages. In the middle ages the scholastics and the Catholic church saw life in mechanistic terms and postulated a first cause, a tradition that went back to both Aristotelian and earlier Greek scholarship. The idealists in the seventeenth, eighteenth, and nineteenth centuries saw the world in terms of mind and a kind of transcendental subjectivity. We in psychiatry have inherited what appears to be the same contradictory western conundrum, and many physicians have a certain contempt for mind as a psychological frame of observation and reference despite its self-evident presence. Banks, Present, and Steiner (1983) clearly indicated their objections to any consideration of emotional conflict when they said that colitis patients "have been labeled with a wide variety of psychiatric diagnoses. Patients and their families have experienced much unnecessary guilt and anxiety because of the myth that Crohn's disease and ulcerative colitis are 'psychosomatic diseases'" (p. 131). A recent and very questionable study of "psychiatric factors" relating to ulcerative colitis (North, Clouse, Spitznagel, and Alpers, 1990), discusses how patients have "suffered through the years not only with their disease but also with the stigma of the 'psychosomatic label' " (p. 974). Such authors forget their scientific background and are willing to share a prejudice with certain small segments of the community at large. It is an unwarrented prejudicial judgement of the mind.

With a misplaced morality, some members of the public and many physicians seem to feel that one is guilty and personally irresponsible if his or her illness is attributed to psychological causes. But the individual is innocent of guilt-ridden sin if his illness is defined in mechanical organic terms. The poor patient with a "physical" illness is seen as victimized by outside or inherited demons such as germs, accidents, or defective genes. Something or someone else is the villain and the patient is "not guilty" and need not be ashamed. This is characteristic of childlike reasoning and infantile concepts of responsibility. Such prejudiced thought processes in a scientific paper is not only open to question, it is totally unscientific. It is a semantic error.

It is fascinating that such a moral stance is adopted by so many investigators, since these same observers also depreciate the subjective and pronounce their mechanistic, organic physical observations as the *only* scientific approach, in which the data are evaluated as an intellectually elevated position. Their view of science does not include any other areas of observation, despite the obvious subjectivity of themselves as observers. Consensual validation of subjective data is apparently meaningless to them because it involves subjective observations. A whole body of observable coordinate scientific material is denied and overlooked.

Let us now consider Freud's *mysterious leap* and David Graham's designation of *independence* and *interactionism* (1967).

As an empiricist I have to agree with the physician Almy in his description of psychosomatic illness as a parallel construct (1975):

The term psychosomatic is here used to describe any reaction of the organism to environmental stress in which objective bodily changes and emotional disturbances occur in parallel. . . . This concept implies a biological response of the organism as a whole, an arousal of its general defensive reaction pattern, even though it may appear to be concentrated in the function of a single organ, such as the colon. *It denies that the emotions themselves cause bodily changes*—they are merely the affective features of the total reaction [pp. 37–38].

Here an internist and physiologist describes psychosomatic illness in what is an empirically demonstrable fashion. Although he talks about disease, I shall extend his parallelism to a concept of mind and body as general propositions in both health and disease. Recognition of parallel data bases often involves simultaneity, wherein we can infer or conclude an identity. In Almy's presentation, the identity is, of course, the demonstrated disease process which may be described from the patient's subjective point of view or from the physician's description of physical changes.

I don't feel that any medical observer could disagree with the concept that any thought, idea, or emotion is simultaneously accompanied by cerebral activity, neuronal transmission, synaptic connections, and neurophysiological processes. Most investigators would agree with the inference of identity between mind and brain. Unless we ignore the temporal inferences inherent in causality we cannot say that the neuronal processes cause the thought, idea, or emotion. Thoughts or emotions do not cause neurophysiological activity, nor does neurophysiology cause emotional or thought patterns. Both are simultaneous and these rather simple psychological and physiological facts are empirically demonstrable. We have parallel simultaneous observations.

LINGUISTICS AND CAUSALITY

Graham's (1967) position was "medical, but this does not appear to involve any loss of generality. Medicine offers a specific example of a broad problem" (p. 52).

Independence refers to what amounts to a radical duality of mind and body. In this concept, mind is a separate entity or "thing" from body as it is so often portrayed in the literature of physiology and psychiatry. Thus an illness is either functional or organic. The separation is clear in the description of colitis by Banks, Present, and Steiner (1983, p. 133). Illustrations of independence exist in almost unlimited number in medical literature. For example: "A healthy mind in a healthy body"; and "His condition is not physical, it is all mental." In each case the mind and body are seen as completely separate entities.

Graham clearly illustrates the confusion and contradictions inherent in this differentiation: mental and physical are names of different languages, not of different kinds of events. He notes that his position most closely resembles psychophysiological parallelism: "However, the parallelism lies in the *ways of describing* events, and not in the operation of two mysterious things called 'mind' and 'body' " (p. 57).

The radical separation of what are conceived of as entities, body and mind (body and soul) dates back to the ancients. It was Descartes who most clearly defined "thinking substance" (1637, p. 127; 1644, pp. 208, 210) and "extended substance" (1644, pp. 208, 210) and postulated how they affected and even opposed each other.

This brings us to a second term, *interactionism*, which describes events arising from *independence*, the belief that mind and body are independent entities that interact. We should underline here the materialistic concept of entity.

INTERACTIONISM

Interactionism is the doctrine that mind and body are separate independent entities that cause or affect each other directly.

Freud in his work on aphasia (1891) claimed to adhere to the doctrine of psychophysiological parallelism, but fell into interactionism in 1894 in his paper on the neuro-psychoses of defense. He introduced the crossed-over linear and temporal concept of body to mind and mind to body. Later he referred to the puzzling aspects of that "leap" in his "Notes Upon a Case of Obsessional Neurosis" (1909) and it continued to trouble him throughout his entire career.

Felix Deutsch and Elvin Semrad in their survey of Freud's writings in *On the Mysterious Leap from the Mind to the Body* (1959) say this about Freud's ideas about the relationship of physical and psychological processes:

> Two opinions he has held all his life. One was that there was no evidence of psychical processes occurring apart from physiological ones, and that no mental process could exist apart from a brain [i.e., parallel doctrine]. The other was that physical processes must precede psychical ones, that is, information reaching the mind, whether from the outer world through the sense organs, or from the body through the chemical stimuli it provides, must begin as a physical excitation [pp. 27–28].

Freud's cloudy interactionist doctrine seems to be partially contradicted by his return to an implied parallelistic position in *New Introductory Lectures* (1933a): "what we are talking now is biological psychology, we are studying the psychical accompaniments of biological processes" (pp. 95–96).

Freud was not the only investigator to trip over an interactionist position. Stanley Cobb handled what he considered the problem to be with apparent simplicity (1963) when he recalled: "Twenty years ago at a Lowell Lecture at the Boston Public Library, I said, 'I solved the "mind–body" problem by stating that there is no such problem' " (p. 36). Despite an introductory quote from Feigl (1958), a philosopher who espoused duality of language in the observations of the mind and body, Cobb proceeded, eschewing any serious philosophy or semantics, to explain away dualistic conundrums by an interactionist process of structuring and metaphor (1963): "The monistic philosophy is the only logical one for a medical scientist. . . . When one really accepts monism, one is satisfied with the belief that mind is a process, a product of the brain in action, just as circulation is a process, the result of the heart and vessels in action" (p. 41). He states the same position more tersely: "the brain is the organ of the mind" (p. 42).

Cobb presents an avowed monism with unresolved (and unrecognized) implications. He has adopted an interactionist position with the entity, brain, *causing* mind. He thought he had eliminated duality by placing causality (or "organ of") between the parallel linguistic duality of mind and body.

He also allies himself with many other observers with another definition: "mind is the integration itself, the relationship of one functioning [part of] the living brain to the other functioning parts" (p. 43). Here Cobb makes mind synonymous with organization. This, as Graham (1967) so clearly indicates, is an untenable and contradictory metaphor.

The interactionist proposition that brain is the organ of the mind has been popular with a number of psychoanalysts. It was certainly the way Freud organized his thoughts as he worked on "The Project" (1895). Despite its logical and semantic flaws, it is tempting to utilize the concept as a working hypothesis. As seductive as such a simple formulation may appear, it leads to erroneous mechanical speculations like those in the often-voiced problem of transduction (nerve impulses changing into emotion and vice versa).

Otto Sperling was in substantial agreement with Cobb and so stated (1978a): "In reality I convinced myself early in life that the psyche is the function of the brain" (p. 9).

Charles Brenner, another astute and able psychoanalyst, seemed in agreement when he explained (1982) that "all psychic phenomena are aspects of cerebral functioning" (p. 8). Graham (1967) made pertinent comment on this form and use of "aspects":

[S]uperficially similar statements like, "the mental and physical are two aspects of the same thing," or "mind and body are two sides of the same coin." Our position is that they are not two aspects, but rather two ways of describing the same aspect. "Aspects" refers to *different* observational data, obtained—to take a basic example—by looking at something from two different vantage points. Two sides of a coin obviously yield different data—the "heads" side is different from the "tails" side. Patients can be thought of as having different aspects, but any aspect is suitable for description in the somatic language, and many in the psychological [p. 57].

Parenthetically: Only at this point does Graham use the term and directly consider *data*. While he recognized two separate sources of data on the "two sides of the coin," he does not recognize that the "different observational data" are parallel and may assume an even more significant relevance to the "mind–body" problem "than the parallel nature of the linguistic structures," from the "heads" and "tails" sides. Graham proceeds: "patients can be thought of as having different aspects, but any aspect is suitable for description in the somatic language and many in the psychological" (p. 57).

Engel (1954b) was forthright in admitting difficulties in describing psychosomatic states:

None of the psychosomatic hypotheses so far advanced has fulfilled the requirements both of correctly identifying the somatic process and indicating how psychic processes are related to the somatic. The jump from the psychic phenomena to the physical phenomena at the end organ is conceptually the most difficult and it is impossible to understand without a clear understanding of what can only be expressed in psychologic terms [p. 341].

Engel, wrestling with what he saw as a duality of entities, draws our attention to the contradictions in interactionism, and the reality of linguistic parallelism. He later (1980) became interested in the biopsychosocial approach.

As noted, T. P. Almy conceived of and then rejected the interactionist position and acknowledged parallel observations. He recognized that there may be simultaneity and duality in the frames of observation of the psychiatrist and the physiologist, while each presumably observes the same order of events and each has his own language for his own frame of reference. Almy presented bodily changes and emotional disturbances as parallel propositions but did not follow the semanticists (Korzybski, 1933; Whorf, 1941a,b), the philosopher Feigl (1950, 1958), or the internist Graham (1967) in recognizing separate languages, or coordinates. He did not recognize parallel frameworks of observation, or accumulations of data (Hogan, this chapter).

The complications in our familiar use of interactionism are legion. Alexander (1939) attempted to explain a unity with a duality of observational viewpoints:

> In fact, it becomes obvious that the physiological study of the highest centers of the central nervous system and the psychological study of personality deal with one and the same thing from different points of view. Whereas physiology approaches the functions of the central nervous system in terms of space and time, psychology approaches it in the terms of these subjective phenomena, which we call psychological and they are *subjective reflections of physiological processes* [p. 13].

Despite this approach to a parallelistic concept, his logic falters, and he retreats in a number of places in the same paper to interactionism; mind causing physiology and physiology causing mind.

We can see the contradictions and pitfalls in the interactionist position when we observe Weiner (1977) puzzling over how "perceived social experiences or psychological conflicts and induced emotions can be translated (transduced) into physiological changes leading to disease" (pp. 624–628).

> We do not understand how emotions are translated by efferent neural pathways into physiological changes in the body. And we do not know how afferent neuronal activity, carried in sensory

pathways, acquires psychological meaning and produces emotional responses. The translation from the neural to the psychological must occur twice, and involves a transduction from one form of activity or process to another [p. 625].

Weiner (1977) presents the contradictions clearly, but without resolution when he notes:

Nerve impulses or spikes are quantal phenomena: impulses do not vary with stimulus intensity once the stimulus exceeds threshold. Further, the impulses lack specificity—they are propagated in all axons regardless of origin, by the same mechanism, but with different rates of transmission and different timing [p. 625]. [There is] the conviction that perceived event and the emotional response to it give rise in a causal linear manner to the physiological responses that are controlled by the brain [p. 626].

He even speculates on the possibility "that the presumed causal link may not exist at all: concurrent events are not necessarily causally related" (p. 626).

Weiner proceeds to rather complicated models of transduction without further consideration of the entire concept of causality. He insists on a linear causal process of external perceptions and emotional reactions being "transduced" into neuronal activity. Herein is the greatest indictment of interactionism: the contradictions inherent in the linear and temporal system of causality.

The unrecognized reliance on interactionism and mind–body independence seems to be part and parcel of the psychosomatic literature. Mason (1971), offering some modifications to Selye's (1956) general adaptation syndrome, separates out emotion as a separate entity from the physiological response to stress of "purely physical" nature and notes that "much more subtle psychological stimuli of everyday life can be sensitively reflected in the adrenocortical activity" (p. 325).

Taylor (1987) provides an example of accepting linguistic parallelism and not understanding it at all:

We can bypass the problem of causality and study the mind/
body interface scientifically by adopting Graham's concept of
linguistic parallelism which states that the real difference between
mind and body is not in the events observed but in the languages
and conceptual systems in which they are described. This re-
moves the mind/body problem from the metaphysical plane and
makes it a problem of semantics rather than of causality [p. 172].

He then proceeds to utilize interactionist logic. One of many
examples is Taylor's (1987, p. 279) discussion of Weiner's work
(1970, 1972) when he talks of the possibility that mental and
bodily responses to external stimuli take place over separate
neural pathways. One explicit example of interactionism occurs
when he complains that early psychosomaticists "gave little attention to the *interactional* experiences and neural pathways in
early life that account for the transformation of sensations and
other physiological experiences into psychological representations" (p. 37; emphasis added). Taylor correctly brings our attention to the causality implied in interactionism: mind *causes*
(or synonym) physiology and/or physiology *causes* (or synonym)
mind.

It is important to recognize the temporal factor in causality,
clearly considered and stated by the philosopher Whitehead
(1938): "Consider our notion of 'causation.' How can one event
be the cause of another? In the first place, no event can be
wholly and solely the cause of another event. *The whole antecedent world conspires to produce a new occasion.* But some *one occasion
in an important way conditions the formation of a successor*" (pp.
917–918, emphasis added). "The only intelligible doctrine of
causation is founded on the doctrine of immanence. Each occasion presupposes the antecedent world as active in its own nature" (p. 918).

Parenthetically, it is of interest to note in his definition the
universality of *overdetermination*, one of Freud's contributions
to the understanding of symptom formation. Our immediate
attention is, however, on the temporal sequence in causality,
"antecedent world" (p. 918). We could utilize the definitions of

other philosophers, linguists, or lexicographers, but we would find that, almost universally, they include the idea of temporal sequence, that is, time. Each caused event by definition has an antecedent cause. Any other position would be most unusual.

In the words of that amalgam of cynicism and idealism, the philosopher Bertrand Russell (1929): "The law of causality, I believe, like much that passes muster among philosophers, is a relic of a bygone age, surviving, like the monarchy, only because it is erroneously supposed to do no harm" (p. 387). Despite the temptation to make fun of causality, perhaps even Russell would admit time as a necessary condition for any conceivable law of succession.

In interactionism, therefore, there is a temporal gap between cause and effect, whether one assumes that mind causes physiology or body causes emotion (subdivision of mind, if you will). Weiner (1970, 1972, 1977) and Reiser (1975), when they speculate that mental and bodily responses take place over separate neural pathways, are in error. The concept of transduction of social and personal stimuli into physiological responses is also in error.

Descartes (1575–1650), the most notable proponent of definitions of a radical interactional confrontation of mind and body, saw on the one hand his "thinking substance" (1637, p. 127; 1644, pp. 208, 210) in opposition to his "extended substance" (1644, pp. 208, 213) and on the other hand presented a cause and effect relationship in that the mind comes into contact with the body and influences it with its spirits. He felt that the pineal gland was the major source of the spirits (1629, pp. 100, 106; 1641, p. 59n; 1649, pp. 340–348).

Descartes (1644), in keeping with his time and education, accepted God (p. 210) as the source and organizer of the mind and the body, but many of his contemporaries, while agreeing with him about God, could see the parallel nature of the processes of mind and body. A doctrine of *occasionalism* arose, which accepted the parallel, but proposed that mind and body, like two clocks, were finely attuned to each other in parallel by the hand of God. The argument illustrates the difficulties inherent in the concept of the interaction of parallel "entities," we are actually describing and communicating data from parallel sources, an accumulation allowing us to abstract (and create) identities, events, entities, objects, or however else one wishes to linguistically identify our observations.

PARALLELISM

The parallel nature and simultaneity of observations of mental and physiological observations was shown in T. P. Almy's (1975) attempt to define psychosomatic disease, but our observations, valuations, and interpretations of the parallel data can be complex.

Any investigator should be as interested and informed as to the source, type, and character of the data as to its content. I agree with the observations of Feigl (1950, 1958), Graham (1967), and Freud (1891) that the data we psychiatrists and some neuroscientists deal with presents itself in parallel and often simultaneous forms. It is how we observe and evaluate the relationship of parallel data that is the subject of this chapter.

Traditional parallelism treats the mind and the body as two parallel entities, each separate from the other, but linked by a concept called isomorphism.

Feigl (1950, 1958) and Graham (1967) help us to see that, given the parallel nature of the languages used to describe the mental and the physical (mind and body), we are not dealing with entities but with linguistic styles. Although Graham gave an admirable presentation of parallel linguistics, he did not acknowledge our use of dual and parallel sets of data.

The subject of psychophysiological parallelism is probably best discussed by its moderate critic, Herbert Feigl (1950, 1958) who first proposed linguistic dualism. In 1950 he noted:

[I]f a label is wanted then perhaps "double-language-theory" is still the least misleading I can suggest. . . . This correspondence, however, must not be confused with what is traditionally called psycho-physical or psycho-physiological parallelism. Parallelism has always been a doctrine according to which two different types of processes or two aspects of one and the same process are related by laws of coexistence or contemporaneity [pp. 624–625].

He then added: "Logical Empiricism in its present phase possesses the logical tools for a reformulation of the identity or double-language view of the mental and the physical" (p. 626).

Feigl goes into more detail in his 1958 paper where he contrasts his hypotheses of identity, monism, or dual language to traditional behaviorism, scientific psychology, and, finally, parallelism with isomorphism. In the beginning of the paper he notes, as he discusses those scientific systems of psychological thought predating his dual language proposition or linguistic parallelism, that:

[T]he behaviorist psychologist assimilates his method to that of the "objective" natural sciences. . . . Scientific psychology, as the well known saying goes, having first lost its soul, later its consciousness, seems finally to lose its mind altogether [p. 370].

Feigl describes his dual language theory as a metaphysical doctrine:

Parallelism and isomorphism, now that we have recovered from the excesses of positivism and behaviorism are generally considered as inductively confirmable hypotheses [p. 380]. Psycho-neurophysiological parallelism is here understood as postulating a one-one, or at least a one-many, simultaneity—correspondence between the mental and the physical. Parallelism as customarily conceived clearly rules out a many-one or a many-many correspondence [p. 376].

Feigl points out clearly that the predictability of mental states from neurophysiological states is limited, although the recognition of mental states as existing parallel to neurophysiological states is expected. Having eliminated any interactionism in either parallelism with isomorphism or in dual language parallelism, Feigl proceeds with his argument:

> According to this conception voluntary action as well as psychosomatic processes, such as hysteria, neurotic symptoms, and psychogenic organic disease (e.g., gastric ulcers) may ultimately quite plausibly be explained by the causal effects of cerebral states and processes upon various other parts of the organism; only the cerebral states themselves being correlated with conscious (or unconscious) mental states [pp. 382–383].

In other words, cerebral states parallel conscious or unconscious mental processes. Lines of causality in the physical world may proceed from cerebral functioning and neurophysiology to altered somatic states—the control of the hypothalamo-pituitary-adreno-cortical axis for example—and this causal linkage remains in the observational sphere of the physical. However, it may be compared to and coordinated with the simultaneous observations of data in the parallel realm of ("conscious or unconscious") mental functioning. It is important to recognize that there is no crossover in causality between the physical and the mental (this would be interactionism). The mental introspective world with its conscious or unconscious emotional, symbolic, intellectual, perceptual, or integrative content may reveal its own determinism—causal connections paralleling the physical to a greater or lesser degree. We here include conscious introspection as well as potential or theoretically constructed consciousness when we understand and interpret the unconscious.

Feigl recognizes the parallel orders of observations, but does not see the observations as dual entities connected by isomorphism, as in traditional psychophysiological parallelism. As a consequence of his recognition that one linguistically or graphically describes, records, and/or communicates observations (in my words, "data") from parallel sources he correctly feels that he can maintain a monistic position of identity with his dual language proposition: there is a language of mind and a language of body.

LINGUISTIC PARALLELISM

Here we find ourselves on firm empirical ground when we follow Graham's (1967) presentation. He acknowledges his debt to Feigl, but proceeds with the medical and not the philosophical arguments.

Graham observes that " 'psychological' and 'physical' (and their synonyms) refer to different ways of talking about the *same* event" (p. 52). He specifically and correctly disposes of interactionism and independence. For the sake of medical clarity he ignores the concept of psychophysical parallelism with isomorphism.

Having observed that " 'psychological' and 'physical' cannot be usefully thought of as referring to different kinds of states of events" (p. 52) and that:

> [D]ifferent languages may be used to describe and discuss exactly the same event . . . "mental" and "physical" are names of different languages, not of different kinds of events . . . the language or system is not a property of the event observed . . . the parallelism lies in the way of describing events, and not in the operation of two mysterious things called "mind" and "body" [pp. 56–57].

Graham makes another distinction:

> Linguistic custom in medicine tends to divide diseases into two principal classes. For one class, the words "mental," "emotional," "functional," and "psychogenic" are used almost interchangeably; for the other, the two common words are "physical" and "organic." The same division is applied also to changes in an organism even when illness is not involved [p. 59].

Graham gives us an indication of the relative convenience of the two languages depending upon the subject described. He creates a splendid example of parallel linguistics:

> John Smith was frightened when he saw the cat.

When the light rays from the cat reached John Smith's retina, various biochemical processes were set up that resulted in the passage of impulses over the optic nerve to the occipital cortex, with activation of sympathetic hypothalamic nuclei, and increased activity in sympathetic nerves to the heart, leading to tachycardia . . . [p. 58].

It is clear that one is dealing with a description of the subjective experience, simultaneously paralleling the language of physiology. In my own work I would characterize such experiences as *data*. Obviously in this case the language of feeling is terser and clearer than the language of physiology. Nevertheless we can see the parallel nature of the material.

Graham proceeds:

Although we have considered simple statements that were almost purely descriptive, without much content of inference or explanation, complex theoretical statements can also be made in either language. For instance: "He is afraid of cats because of an unresolved Oedipus complex"; or "Energy for cardiac contraction is derived from high-energy phosphate bonds" [pp. 58–59].

The example that Graham chooses is of tremendous interest. The first frame of observation involves the mind or emotion. It is a separate field of observation. I would add that he is using separate languages for a separate group of coordinates. Emotion does not flow through neurones (Reiser, 1975; Weiner, 1977; Taylor, 1987). It is part of an event with special qualities observed from the frame of reference of the subjective mental world, and it is described in its own linguistic style.

On the other hand, impulses—in the language of neurophysiology—do go through neurones, leading to tachycardia, all part of the simultaneous physiological observational base recorded by ourselves or our instruments in the specific framework of the physical world. It is a description of a part of the chain of physical events that we recognize is simultaneously accompanying the subjectively observed and described emotion, fear. One cannot escape the obvious: there are two coordinate sets of observations and two coordinate linguistic descriptions. At no time are we logically or empirically justified in assuming the interactionist position—crossing over—of assuming that emotion caused the tachycardia or that the tachycardia caused the emotion. They are simultaneous observations with their own appropriate linguistic (including numerical or graphic) descriptions, recordings, and presentations.

My own contribution is the recognition that we are not only recognizing parallel languages, but are recognizing parallel sources of and sets of data. In this light it is hard to accept Weiner's (1977) concept of transduction: "perceived social experience or psychological conflicts and induced emotions can be translated (transduced) into physiological changes leading to disease. A comprehensive understanding of the extremely complex processes by which the translation of the psychological (the nonmaterial) into the physiological (the material) eludes us still" (pp. 624–625). He has hypothesized a temporal succession of events from the subjective to the physical. In reality there is no temporal "translation." We are only observing data from two distinct frames of observation.

LINGUISTIC PARALLELISM AND DISEASE

When dealing with ideas of illness or pathology, there are some very special problems with the terms *functional* and *organic*. While each is a part of one of two separate languages, spheres of observations, or systems of coordinates, each is commonly utilized to describe not only the disease but the presumed cause. Graham (1967) feels that they "are at best useless concepts and at worst seriously misleading" (p. 52). We may be dealing with a neurosis (traditionally functional) and we may observe the anxiety, phobias, or whatever in the realm of the mind. We also could presumably trace the cortico-hypothalamic-pituitary-adrenocortical axis changes as well as neuronal, synaptic, and tachycardial activity that simultaneously accompany the mental. In the latter sphere of observation we are making physical or organic observations. With our contemporary superficial examination we may not be able to fathom or describe any *structural* changes, so despite our clear-cut observation of what seem to be transient but profound cerebral, neurophysiological, physiological, and biochemical activities and changes, we consider the illness mental and call it "functional." What is perhaps worse, the greatest confusion is in the field of neuroscience, where researchers in neurophysiology believe their research is in psychology or psychiatry and vice versa.

Along with Graham, I have great reservations about the words *functional* and *organic* with their implied definitional restrictions (independence) as well as with their implied etiological significance.

Both Feigl and Graham explained that a pattern of causal relationships can occur within only one field of observation, which might be the subjective, i.e., the mind; alternatively, it might be the field of outside experience that includes the physical, i.e., the body, the brain, and all other external objects and activities.

In our study of inflammatory colon diseases, the patients can be observed from a psychological area of inquiry or from a physical window of investigation.

If I construct a hypothetical structure of dynamic interplay it will not necessarily conform to the subjective life or the physical findings of any particular patient or group of patients.

In the language of the mind (in this case, psychoanalytic thought) one might imagine a subjective experience of severe loss or bereavement precipitating (causing) overwhelming unconscious and conscious rage. This in turn leads to (causes) intolerable anxiety, which in turn necessitates (causes) defensive fantasies of denial. These dynamic factors are accompanied by the subjective experience of pain, cramps, and the sensation of colonic evacuation, all symptoms characteristic of colitis.

These subjective activities are paralleled by (and are perhaps simultaneous with) potentially observable activities of the nervous system and gut. As we perceive these coordinated processes we (usually without much conscious thought) assume an identity. Using traditionally interactionist thought patterns we are sometimes prone to contradict ourselves, ignore the identity, and conclude that the activities of the colon are the cause of the patient's discomfort. We are often inclined to ignore the parallel nature of the observations. There are no causal crossovers between the parallel areas of observation.

Coordinated with the subjective world imagined above, one can imagine the physical world where cortical activity sends messages by neurones to initiate (cause) complicated activities of the extended nervous system. These, in turn, possibly lead to (cause) complex activities in the gut.

We must recognize that, in our discussions about, and observations of, the physical world, we are not limited to the brain and the body. That world can include mathematics, physics, and the anatomy of elephants.

PARALLEL SOURCES OF DATA AND LINGUISTIC PARALLELISM

Neither Feigl nor Graham semantically perceived anything beyond parallel linguistic concerns. Both repeatedly worked with "body" and "mind" as irreducible entities with which one must relate and toward which one must accommodate oneself. Graham (1967) had some feeling for the incongruities of the accepted semantic use of the words. I have already noted his statement "parallelism lies in the *ways of describing events*, and not in the operation of two mysterious things called 'mind' and 'body' " (p. 57). Despite the seeming recognition that one is referring only to nouns (those "things"), Graham proceeds to confirm his certainty of their existence, in disagreement with Feigl: he and Feigl seem to label—what I would designate as a "source of data"—an avenue to knowledge. Graham argues that "[Feigl] later suggested that 'two avenues to knowledge' would be a better designation. The position of the present essay is that even when there is only one avenue to knowledge, the choice of two languages remains" (p. 57).

It is clear that Graham separates his linguistic parallelism from any "avenue to knowledge."

Neither Feigl nor Graham took the extra step from their monumental discoveries of "dual language theory" and "linguistic parallelism" to the recognition that mind and body are not irreducible "things" (Graham, 1967, p. 57), or irreducible entities. "Mind" and "body" are words, nouns representing accumulations of data in space and time.

Even if one ignores the very important semantic "frills," it should be apparent to any scientific investigator that while one may be working with a labeled entity, i.e., the body, one is at the same time working with a potentially immense amount of diverse data: the appearance of the body, the nervous system, the pathology observable after the body's terminal illness, and theoretical formulations relating to the various categories of data. Each category is an abstraction of data from a particular frame of observation. While our abstractions and labels (one could say "files") are useful, each is an amalgam of data, contemporary or historical.

The same principles apply to that parallel "entity" or label, the mind. One's subjective data can be as diverse as that of a colleague investigating the anatomy of the body that "mind" is a file of subjective material: the emotions, cognition, impulses, defenses, and theories about subjective psychological and psychiatric worlds.

I like the nondefinitional term *event* as a description of an object, a point in time, or an activity in progress. *Event* can lose its value if it is used only as a metaphor for an irreducible labeled entity (Graham, 1967). It is only when we play around with such labels for accumulations of data that we find ourselves embroiled in a mind–body problem. There are two separate parallel sources of data in nature, in which the data are concerned with nature itself; unfortunately, they are often recognized now as the mind and the body. We have to cast aside such erroneous assumptions and understand that there are no irreducible "independent" entities "interacting" or existing in parallel with another label (word), *isomorphism*, utilized as a conceptual bridge between two parallel "entities."

Chapter 8
Mind, Language, and Organization

LANGUAGES AND ORGANIZATION

DIFFERENT LANGUAGES AND SUBLANGUAGES

Both Feigl (1950, 1958) and Graham (1967) make the point that under the concept of mind we may have a number of sublanguages, of which one is psychoanalysis. In many sublanguages we recognize that linguistic styles are divided according to the level of abstraction. For example, in a psychoanalytic investigation a description of a specific sadistic erotic fantasy, its determinants, its effects, and the defenses against it is obviously at a much lower level of abstraction than is a metapsychological discussion of the superego and its general responses to primitive impulses.

I think some of the arguments about drive derivatives as opposed to object relations might be better understood if we admitted different levels of abstraction.

The physical, too, has many different sublanguages such as anatomy, physiology, biochemistry, and molecular biology. Each of these physical sublanguages has subsublanguages with their own levels of abstraction.

As Graham (1967) said, "Speakers can be right or wrong in either language" (p. 58); "Neither language or system is intrinsically more correct or scientific than the other language or system" (p. 57); "[F]inding one language useful in no way excludes

81

the use of others" (p. 59). The utilization of one language, system of coordinates, or sphere of observation does not invalidate any other framework of observation or investigation. The task in psychosomatic medicine is to find a dictionary that allows us closer and closer approximations of meanings between languages. In my words: The understanding of and coordination between sets of data from parallel sources of data is the constant work at hand.

We can use languages other than the mental or physiological. In the "objective" world we can see that sociology, epidemiology, and behaviorism each has a language of its own and each has its own orders of abstraction. Their languages are in the realm of the physical world; epidemiology, sociology, and behaviorism seem to have more in common with the physiological languages of the body than they do with the language of the mind.

To illustrate the careful linguistic separation of data, consider observations of infants by the psychoanalyst Mahler (1967). For the most part her investigation of children is not observation of the psyche nor is it per se psychoanalytic. It is observation of behavior and physiology and is appropriately communicated in the descriptive language of the physical; the data should be recognized as stemming from such observations. However, here the word *leap* is appropriate: As the investigator is willing to leap backward from the subjective associations of older children and adults, he is able to infer coordinates rich with meaning.

Studies like Mahler's offer psychoanalysts behavioristic and physical dimensions to supplement reconstructed subjective content, and establish relative verification as we interpret reconstructions in older children and adults that open new memories or eliminate symptoms.

Other scientists and writers have delved into the subject of linguistic expression. The linguist Whorf (1941a) notes: "Every language and every well-knit technical sublanguage incorporates certain points of view and certain patterned resistances to widely divergent points of view" (p. 247). He also wisely observes (1941b) that: " 'thinking is a matter of LANGUAGE' is an incorrect generalization of the more nearly correct idea that 'thinking is a matter of different tongues' " (p. 239).

Korzybski (1933) describes the nature of linguistic communication: "The object *is not words.* . . . The object is absolutely unspeakable because no amount of words will make the object" (p. 226).

If we speak of a human event, thought, or body part in either subjective psychological terms (from one observational viewpoint) or in physical organic terms (another viewpoint), we are utilizing the words of a language to describe the data that define the event, thought, or body part. If the abstraction representing such event, thought, or body part is not visibly at hand, the words make it so! It is interesting to recognize the psychological progression from preverbal to verbal, and to realize that there may be a very early subjective experience of identity of the human event, thought, or body part with the words used to describe it. The event, thought, or body part takes on greater and greater dimensions of meaning as our areas of observation multiply and widen—anatomy, microbiology, linguistics, semantics.

Mind as Organization

Some authors have felt it necessary to place mind somewhere on a physical continuum with body or assume that mind is in some way a matter of organization of the physical parts of the brain. Many try to place mind at the top of an anatomical or physiological hierarchy. At times this amounts to a literal positioning of mind on *top* of the brain. Verbal constructions and metaphor are often used to justify such explanations, which might be an attempt to preserve what is presented as a monist and sometimes materialistic concept. In either case there is an error. A duality does exist—not necessarily a duality of events or entities, but a duality of spheres of observation, of fields of investigation, of coordinates or of linguistic presentations, whichever way one wishes to express it.

Among many examples of avowed monists we have Cobb (1963) who claimed that "mind is the integration itself, the relationship of one functioning part of the living brain to the other functioning parts" (p. 43).

Mason (1971) explains that the "distinction between a 'behavioral' versus a 'physiological' concept is not intended to imply, of course, any fundamental biological difference between psychological and other physiological functions, but simply to call attention to the important question of the *level* within the central nervous system . . ." (p. 331). He not only sees psychological and physiological in terms of levels in the nervous system but goes on to equate psychological with both hierarchical levels and with organization.

Other examples of hierarchies of neurological and psychological entities are legion. Since so many illustrations are available in the medical literature, I shall not burden the reader further. Please note that I do not specifically fault the work of the authors mentioned. Any number of other examples from equally distinguished authors would have served.

Many philosophers conceive of mind as part of a neurological hierarchy. John Searle, an expert on minds and computers, in his six Reith Lectures on *Minds, Brains and Science* (1984) gives us innumerable illustrations: "Now, because mental states are features of the brain, they have two levels of description—a higher level in mental terms, and a lower level in physiological terms. . . . The mind and the body interact but they are not two different things, since mental phenomena just are features of the brain" (p. 26). And: "So within the neurophysiological level there will be a series of levels of description, all of them equally neurophysiological. Now in addition to this, there will also be a mental level of description" (p. 54). Searle here defines the mind as an entity spatially oriented above the brain, but an entity also defined by the complexity of its organization.

Mind is an entity neither spatially placed above brain nor in a hierarchy of levels in the nervous system. Nor is it a separate entity, differentiated from brain only by the complexity of its organization.

PSYCHE AND SOMA

Just as there is no temporal distance between mind and body, there is certainly no spatial distance. Mind is not a superattenuated structure fastened to the top of the brain.

We know that the observation of mind and body are parallel observations and we utilize parallel languages to describe the data. One should not worship the mind to such an extent that one insists that the *complexity of its organization* is what differentiates it from body (brain). But many scientists seem to approach mind with just this overidealization.

Dualistic arguments about man and universe go back before the sixth century B.C. in Greece when theology came into conflict with observation (Thales, 636–546 B.C.); while Pythagoras (582–507 B.C.) combined the two. Plato (427?–547? B.C.) had his soul and Aristotle (384–322 B.C.) his organization. The battle between solipsism and stoicism is as old as whenever man conceived of mind and brain, subjective and objective. Since the Renaissance a battle has raged in the western world between scholasticism and idealism.

The mathematician, René Descartes, is commonly associated with radical dualism. Actually Descartes (1644, pp. 208, 210) in searching for a starting place became interested in his own consciousness and made his argument, "Cogito, ergo sum" (I think, therefore I exist) (1637, p. 127). From there he reasoned that since he could conceive of perfection and God, both must exist. His faith was in the subjective and he was an idealist. He separated existence into his "thinking substance" (1644, pp. 208, 210) and "extended substance" (1637, p. 127; 1644, pp. 208, 210). In so doing he separated reality into two substances, but at the same time did his best to explain all the world (except God and his soul) with mathematical laws. His was a philosophy anchored in doubt, but which included a subjective surety of his own existence. Nevertheless his separation of mind and body as opposing but interacting entities has codified the concepts of independence and interactionism.

I have already referred to the semantics of Korzybski (1933) that contribute a great deal to our understanding of the problems of abstractions and the purely descriptive nature of words, but little to the solution of the mind–body problem. I should mention Whorf (1941a,b) whose brilliance in proposing the idea that fact and reality are only demonstrable in languages is not directly pertinent to our discussion.

Alfred North Whitehead saw words as the communication of data about events, entities, or identities. The journalist Price (1954) quotes Whitehead warning us about words: "*The mistake is to think of words as entities* [emphasis added]. They depend for their force, and also for their meaning, on emotional associations and historical overtones, and derive much of their effect from the impact of the whole passage in which they occur" (p. 229).

Unfortunately, many scientists automatically considered the word the entire entity, and equated the presumed entity with the word. Following this line of reasoning, the entity is often "scientifically" divided into smaller entities that are equated with descriptive words. There is no recognition that one is dealing with data and abstractions of data. Thought becomes fragmented and particularized. Whorf observed (1941b) that "segmentation of nature is an aspect of grammar—one as yet little studied by grammarians. We cut up and organize the spread and flow of events . . . By these more or less distinct terms we ascribe a semifictitious isolation to parts of experience" (p. 240).

For the moment, let us consider Freud and his intuitive understanding of the apparent complex duality of mind and body. Here I want to underline his intuitive knowledge and use of language. The Goethe prize in 1930 is enough of an endorsement of his skills at linguistic communication—his art. He held two positions—one of psychophysiological parallelism and the other of causal interactionism (the mysterious leap). For all this, he brilliantly and intuitively recognized linguistic parallelism. When Freud gave up "The Project" (1895) he recognized the impossibility of abstracting his observations and ideas of and about the psyche in the language of neurophysiology. He decided to utilize psychological terms and descriptions to present his psychological observations and conclusions. Here, without elaborating the principle, he utilized parallel positions linguistically.

He recognized the need for different frames of reference (spheres of observation or sublanguages) in order to present the different dimensions of his observations. In "The Unconscious" (1915) he developed what he termed his "metapsychology," defining the topographical point of view (pp. 172–173) and the economic and dynamic: "I propose that when we have succeeded in describing a psychical process in its dynamic, topographical and psychic aspects we should speak of it as a *metapsychological* presentation" (p. 181).

It would be difficult to argue with the proposition that at this point Freud acknowledged the need to look at a given event from a number of points of view (observational frames of reference, all within the framework of mind). In each case he utilized a new and different language. He added another new sublanguage, his structural theory (1923) of id, ego, and superego without apology, not indicating that his theory in any way contradicted earlier assertions but further clarified psychic activity as he saw it. In some ways his structural theory was a different order of abstraction from his earlier work.

One could make the argument that such intuitive use of what Graham described as linguistic parallelism—with sublanguages for psychic abstractions—was among the most important contributions to the clarity of Freud's expositions.

The separation between his linguistic metapsychology and the subjective experience was always clear. A psychic event could be described from the point of view of specific psychic content and conflict or from a more abstract psychoanalytic or metapsychological stance. Each description was in a separate language and often on a separate level of abstraction. Neither necessarily contradicted nor excluded the other.

Freud was far too concerned with the lucid presentations of his clinical discoveries to allow himself any preoccupation with his methods of presentation. Despite his assurances that he had given up philosophy as a fruitless endeavor, he indicates his recognition of linguistic structure and perhaps acknowledges a philosophical interest in his *New Introductory Lectures* (1933a): "The theory of the instincts is so to say our mythology. Instincts are mythical entities, magnificent in their indefiniteness. In our work we cannot for a moment disregard them, yet we are never sure that we are seeing them clearly" (p. 95). In his September 1932 letter to Einstein (1933b) Freud again addressed this linguistic problem in his own way, referring to the death instinct. "It may perhaps seem to you as though our theories are a kind of mythology and, in the present case, not even an agreeable one. But does not every science come in the end to a kind of mythology like this? Cannot the same be said to-day of your own Physics?" (p. 211).

Nevertheless, in these sublanguages of psychoanalysis, his metapsychological abstractions, he presented us with a view of psychological activity from a number of spheres of observation; recognizing that each was within the framework of mind, of subjective experience, and of conscious and unconscious motivation.

Although, in practice, he did not always follow his early avowed doctrine of simultaneous parallelism, allowing himself to be caught in the dilemma of the mysterious leap, he certainly was more than successful in evolving languages for various simultaneous points of view. For the most part in Freud's writing there was no doubt as to the clear separation between his linguistic psychology and the event which could be viewed from a number of psychoanalytic points of view. Also, for the most part, there was a clear definition between the psychoanalytic and the physical presentation of the event. He did seem to return to parallelism in "The Theory of Instincts" (1933a): ". . . what we are talking now is biological psychology, we are studying the psychical accompaniments of biological processes" (p. 95). The main exceptions to such a clear definition were in some of his longer theoretical treatises such as "Beyond the

Pleasure Principle" (1920) and "Group Psychology and the Analysis of the Ego" (1921).

The physician George Groddeck (1912, 1923, 1977) was among the most brilliant of the early clinicians to puzzle over the accuracy of semantic presentation. This modest but intellectually imperious physician demonstrated in his chapter on language (1912) his knowledge of words and reality, primarily with his linguistic nihilism. He indicated his intuitive grasp of the profound error of assuming the identity of language with the object or event that is described. He notes: "Language has created religion and art, built streets and conducted trade all over the world. . . . Agriculture is as unthinkable without language as is philosophy . . . God and nature are dependent on language" (p. 248). Here he not only describes language but also indicates man's use of it for creation as well as communication. However, he goes on to complain about "the culturally inhibiting effects of language, the invincible claims by which language enslaves our thought and action. There is the well-known saying that man was given language in order to hide his thoughts. . . . Man's most personal thought is speechless" (p. 249). Despite his disparagement of language he states most eloquently: "We speak of a piece of bread, a glass of water, a picture, a star, as if they were self-contained objects with defined frontiers. This is wrong. They do not exist as separate objects, we do not perceive of them as separate" (p. 250). Groddeck comments on science with a real understanding of various frames of observation. "This is how one should go about doing research. Grip the object in front of you tightly, look at it and touch it on all sides, yet when you have done that remember that this apparent whole is merely a part, a dependent link in a chain" (p. 251).

After displaying initial interest, Groddeck refused to identify himself with traditional psychoanalysis, despite Freud's admiration for his work and their prolonged correspondence. Much of Groddeck's refusal had to do with his mistrust of any verbal theoretical formulations, his distrust of linguistic conclusions as representations of truth: "We are barbarians, yet we have the possibility of producing a genuine culture in future. But language, the most important tool with which to further this, almost entirely fails us. Perhaps other means will appear later which are more useful for the spirit and for truth" (1912, p. 264).

I cannot imagine what Groddeck had in mind when he mentioned "other means," but perhaps we can better define and describe the truth when we can utilize multiple languages for multiple frames of observation, relieving us of our perceived dependence on Aristotelian causality with the excluded third (Korzybski, 1933) as well as our misapprehension that brain causes mind or mind causes brain. With such a recognized multiplicity of sources of data, we might even satisfy part of Groddeck's need for a more genuine culture with less barbarity.

Groddeck recognized what the semanticists later attempted to examine: language is always a tentative tool for explaining the data of reality—or perhaps we should say presenting the data of what we perceive this day, to be reality. But language did allow him to communicate his observations on the relativity of "facts." He discerned, but did not describe, the multiplicity of points of observation (languages) necessary to come closer to truth and fact. We might even approach Whorf's goal of recognizing the relativity and relationships of the facts of science (1941a). We are at least aware that words are not entities as Whitehead observed (Price, 1954, p. 229), and that "the object is not words. . . . The object is unspeakable because no amount of words will make the object (Korzybski, 1933, p. 226).

Chapter 9
Conversion Reaction

Theory of Conversion

Clinically, one of the most productive concepts in the realm of psychoanalysis has been Freud's formulation of hysterical conversion (1894, 1909). If we briefly review the background we see that, despite Freud's proclaimed parallelistic thinking (1891, 1933a), he indicated his bewilderment about the relation between the mind and the body proposing the "mysterious leap," an interactionist concept of causality. He differentiated between what in this context he saw as two entities, mind and body, which interact. There is a temporal gap implied in such interaction and causality. The leap has also been used to describe the opposite: body causing mind.

Deutsch (1922) by implication broadened the term *conversion* to include pregenital determinants. But he, too, had trouble recognizing the separation of parallelism from interactionism and in understanding the isomorphic aspects of traditional parallelism. "Whatever the cause may be, the concept of psychophysical parallelism must be rejected, for nothing parallel occurs here. The temporal coincidence of psychic and physical manifestations develops from the identity of these processes" (1922, p. 69). At that time the idea of parallelism and isomorphic parallelism did exist, but the concept of linguistic parallelism had not been offered to the medical world; the recently introduced recognition of parallel sources of data was just as unknown. We could agree that the "identity" in the latter part of Deutsch's statement is probably true. But he did not recognize that if we assume an identity we have to base that assumption on parallel sets of simultaneous data. Whether we organize the data with the awkward concept of isomorphism to explain two sources of information about what appear to be two identical processes, or with the recognition of linguistic parallelism, we are dealing with identifiable simultaneous parallel data which may well represent an identity of process.

Deutsch here (1922) seems to violate his perception of identity and simultaneity and indulge in interactionist causality: "The transitory feeling of tension occurs with the transmission of the hormonal product of the germ cells into all cell units, a condition which finally calls for the discharge of the generated energy" (p. 70). And much later (1959) the identity (or parallelistic) theme is contradicted: "Impulses of any quality, chemical or neurogenic, lead to electrical stimulation and produce sensations that are mental constituents par excellence" (p. 93). Here the faulty interactionism between neurogenic impulses and "mental constituents" of sensation is clear. The temporal causal succession is evident. Deutsch's comments indicate how one has to become involved in juggling complicated, often contradictory, explanations if there is not a clear recognition that the investigator is without question dealing with a duality of simultaneous observations when recording or presenting identity in psychosomatic (mind–body) phenomena. Only with this recognition can we understand psychosomatic unity as opposed to two separate existing entities separated by time or space. It is the only way of acknowledging Deutsch's "identity."

Deutsch did see that pregenital determinants coincided with physiological changes in psychosomatic states. Here he extended Freud's formulation of the "leap" of hysteria to a "leap" from unconscious preoedipal conflict to the vegetative nervous system, bodily internal organs, and general physiology. He and Semrad (Deutsch and Semrad, 1959) noted that Freud, "in his paper 'From the History of an Infantile Neurosis' (1918 [1914]) points out that the conversion process may also involve the visceral organs. The unconscious repressed homosexuality withdrew into his big bowel" (p. 35). Deutsch's idea of "organ" conversion states were based on (accompanying) pregenital conflicts and fantasies.

Fenichel (1945b) introduced the term *pregenital conversion.* He noted that conversion symptoms can involve the vegetative nervous systems, but he also felt that not all somatic symptoms of a psychogenic nature should be called conversion because not all were *translations* of specific fantasies into a body language. But one might question Fenichel's use of the word *translation.* Doesn't translation imply time and causality?

To return to the evolution of Freud's own thought on the coining of the term *conversion* we find that in Freud's "Project for a Scientific Psychology" (1895) he made his final attempt to describe psychological mechanisms in the language of neurophysiology. Then he recognized his need for a psychological language in order to present the functions of the mind. He had an avid interest in formulating an energic description for psychic phenomena, an approach that still seemed to utilize the same reasoning as in his physiological work. His alliance with nineteenth-century determinism was strong.

The question has already been discussed from various points of view (Holt, 1967; Gill, 1976). Freud's interest was in the transfer of energy (Breuer and Freud, 1893–1895):

> It is impossible any longer at this point to avoid introducing the idea of quantities (even though not measurable ones). We must regard the process as though a sum of excitation impinging on the nervous system is transformed into chronic symptoms in so far as it has not been employed for external action in proportion to its amount. Now we are accustomed to find in hysteria that a considerable part of this 'sum of excitation' of the trauma is transformed into purely somatic symptoms. . . .
> If, for the sake of brevity, we adopt the term 'conversion' to signify the transformation of psychical excitation into chronic somatic symptoms . . . [p. 86]. [And again,] "The hysterical method of defence—for which, as we have seen, the possession of a particular proclivity is necessary—lies in the conversion of the excitation into a somatic innervation" (p. 122).

Here we can see the evolution of Freud's thought as he lent temporal qualities to his evolving concept of psychic energy, an extension or a recapitulation of his ideas of nervous energy.

Breuer was willing to give credit for the term *conversion* to Freud. In "On the History of the Psycho-Analytic Movement" (1914) Freud noted that "whenever Breuer, in his theoretical contribution to *The Studies on Hysteria* (1895), referred to this process of conversion, he always added my name in brackets after it. . . ." Breuer later accepted partial credit. Perhaps we can understand his reluctance better if we recognize how he held out for what was essentially a parallelistic position in linguistic terms (Breuer and Freud, 1893–1895):

> In what follows little mention will be made of the brain and none whatever of molecules. Psychical processes will be dealt with in the language of psychology; and, indeed, it cannot possibly be otherwise. . . . For while ideas are constant objects of our experience and are familiar to us in all their shades of meaning, 'cortical excitations' are on the contrary rather in the nature of a postulate, objects which we hope to be able to identify in the future. . . . I may perhaps be forgiven if I make almost exclusive use of psychological terms [p. 185].

Breuer goes on to describe what is essentially his parallelistic concept of the processes involved. He does not directly contradict Freud's energic constructions or the leap from psyche to the soma but ignores them. Perhaps Breuer took less interest in "The Project" than was previously suspected.

PREGENITAL CONVERSION

The concept of pregenital conversion has played an extremely important role in the psychoanalytic descriptions of psychosomatic disorders. I have already called attention to Deutsch's, Fenichel's, and Semrad's interest. Cecil Mushatt (1954, 1959, 1975, 1989) repeatedly utilized and evolved the concept. Melitta Sperling (1963, 1973) found the formulation of great value in her successful treatment of psychosomatic patients. Otto Sperling (1978a) emphasizes: "If the psychoanalyst adheres to these principles the treatment of psychosomatic disease is not much different from the treatment of conversion hysteria" (p. 7), and he has utilized the idea of pregenital conversion repeatedly. C. P. Wilson (1983a, 1989e) found pregenital conversion a practical way of viewing psychosomatic problems and notes (1989e): "asthma, like other psychosomatic symptoms, is a pregenital conversion symptom" (p. 348). Sarnoff (1989) has given us an interesting developmental formulation of symbolization and symptom formation.

McDougall (1989) classifies psychosomatic phenomena as "archaic hysteria" and seems to accept the concept of pregenital conversion but feels that:

[The psychological meanings are of a] presymbolic order, in that they are the result of a primitive attempt to deal with what we might well term psychotic anxieties. . . . [N]either psychotic nor neurotic symptoms have been created to compensate for what has been ejected from consciousness, because the anxieties aroused have been unable to achieve a mental representation in a symbolic, verbal (i.e., thinkable) form [p. 55].

Despite the semantic critique to follow, I too have found the concept useful and historically meaningful, both in "hysterical conversion syndromes" and "pregenital conversion states." Whenever I found a somatic symptom paralleling a fantasy dramatized in the symptom it seemed appropriate to make use of the traditional language.

I feel that if we use the term *conversion* for symptoms involving striated musculature which ordinarily in healthy circumstances seem to be under conscious (cerebral) control, we have every right to use the term *pregenital conversion* as a term for symptoms involving organs less obviously under conscious (cerebral) control, but organs that in their dysfunction parallel derivatives of pregenital fantasies having to do with subjective perceptions of that organ or its use. Such concomitant psychological reactions frequently involve smooth muscle, the autonomic nervous system, general physiology, biochemical processes, and organ systems.

Technically and linguistically there is no interactionism between mind and body; mind does not cause the physical nor does the physical cause the mind. There may be a temporal sequence of causality in the activity of the central nervous system, its neurophysiological and its physiological connections; and in a parallel way there may be a temporal progression, with causality, in the activity of the psychological sphere. As we have just seen, similar observations were made by Breuer (1893–1895). The observation that a fantasy is simultaneous with correlate physical reaction *does not represent cause* however much our conventional manner of thinking wants to phrase it that way. The two occurring as contemporaneous data may allow the fantasy to be expressed verbally, and the organ symptom to disappear, but the simultaneity rules out causality. We might say that one (fantasy or physical symptom) *represents* the other (physical symptom or fantasy). The data of one are the coordinate of the data of the other. Treatment directed at the modification of one, if successful, may be accompanied by data indicating modification of the parallel "other."

Unfortunately, even with my continued use of the term, I am stuck with the recognition that the term *conversion* literally means converting from psyche to soma and implies a time relationship and differential between the psyche and soma as the "leap" or transfer occurs between the two—*we all know that it takes time to jump*, if only a moment.

However, the term *conversion* is so well established that I cannot foresee any important immediate changes in the use of it, so I shall continue to comply, with the understanding that I am using it only in its historical sense.

I defer my discussion of symbol formation in conversions until part III, the psychoanalytic treatment of inflammatory disease of the colon (see chapter 13). I anticipate myself here by suggesting that in the preverbal and early verbal periods of life the splitting of affect from content in subjective infantile experiences seems to be ubiquitous and allows for a pattern of fragmentation, isolation, and denial. The extent of the denial and repression of split-off ego fragments varies with the extent of the pathology of development. Mind you, this idea of pathology acknowledges hereditary vulnerabilities and predispositions as well as subjective responses to traumatic situations, stimuli, and environments.

McDougall (1982a, p. 84; 1985, p. 174) discusses her concept of the processes of splitting and projective identification that she feels are set in motion to protect the patient from primitive fantasies and feelings. I cannot quite agree with her further description (1985) that "affective perceptions are largely eliminated and with them goes the destruction of meaning. Feeling is not disavowed, it no longer exists" (p. 84). Or where she notes (1985) that "they have split off from consciousness large segments of their psychic reality, thereby expelling a series of fantasies or emotions in order not to feel them" (p. 174). The description is dramatic and informative, but does seem to carry some minor contradictions. If, for instance, the fantasies are literally expelled (no longer in fantasy) where do they go? They go wherever they would no longer be available for potential recognition because there could be no recovery of an eliminated or expelled fantasy or affect in later treatment. My only real disagreement with McDougall is that the fantasies and/or emotion are split off and repressed—often with an accompanying fantasy of expulsion. They do not, however, disappear. They remain in the unconscious and/or preconscious. They may become available for conscious recognition with successful psychoanalytic treatment and the resolution of the psychopathology. There has been no literal expulsion.

A brief description of the context (ego state) in which the primitive antecedents to the later pregenital conversions are formed is summarized in Lewin's comment (1950): "The unconscious meaning of an event depends on its past history, and the infantile prototype is usually altered by the processes of development" (p. 135).

I do not feel that the recognition of ego states in any way contradicts our recognition that symbolization and fantasy can contemporaneously accompany a symptom. As a matter of fact, a split-off ego state would seem to help in the denial and repression of the original affective state, ego state, and whatever subjective fantasy life accompanied such feeling states. When dealing with psychosomatic difficulties we recognize that many subjective experiences must have been preverbal and had to be translated at a later date into words by either the patient or analyst. Over time, feelings, as Lewin (1950) noted, accumulate different levels of content (fantasy).

Once one recognizes that psyche always parallels soma, one must assume a subjective life of the infant even at earliest stages of development. Many psychologists and psychoanalysts have erroneously postulated a prepsychological physiological period of development. That this subjective experience may be preverbal and difficult to translate into postverbal concepts does not limit either its existence or limit the possibility of translation.

Clinical vignette: A psychosomatic patient of mine, trying to find words for his feelings of shame and depression, which somehow went along with a feeling of deprivation, was surprised by a sensation of intense anger. He developed a new acute transient symptom. His masseter muscles went into spasm and he could not open his jaw. That night he dreamed of atomic disintegration of planets in space. He and I had little difficulty in recognizing the postverbal expression of preverbal rage in the transient hysterical symptom and the dream. The rage's relationship to oral conflicts was obvious, and seemed to be confirmed when an area of repressed material, derived from an intermediate level of development, was opened to memory—surrounding the birth of a sister when he was 2½ years of age. Further analysis seemed to confirm that the repression and denial were facilitated by a split in which sadistic contemptuous and destructive fantasies about the primary part object representations were repressed and denied when subjected to reaction formations, splitting, and projective identifications.

I include this example to demonstrate that we are dealing not only with a repressed infantile fantasy, but also with constantly utilized dynamic defensive systems in which contemporary split-off and denied sadism will be found associated with sadistic responses at each and every developmental phase. Very early primitive sadism (fantasies and affect) that has been handled by splitting and denial seems to contribute to splitting and denial whenever an individual experiences intense aggression. In a similar vein, defenses against destructive impulses, from the most primitive to the most sophisticated, may be observed at each level of development. Whether or not the accompanying physiological symptomatology takes on secondary psychological elaborations (Reiser, 1975, 1978; L. Deutsch, 1980) is relatively unimportant. I doubt whether any affective experience does not connect itself with additional layers of content as the individual matures. An adult does not verbalize or think about an oedipal fantasy or memory in the language of an oedipal child. The same observation is true for preoedipal fantasies or memories.

Let me create a scenario artificially isolating an affect associated intimately with psychosomatic patients and early development. The affect is shame or humiliation. Clinical experience teaches us that shame and/or humiliation is first associated with the confusion of affect concerned with oral needs, the mother, and the breast, and may reappear throughout life to a lesser or greater extent when one is denied an expected gratification. The humiliation is apparently accompanied in infancy by the precursors of rage and the wish for (and perhaps one may assume hallucination of) omnipotent control. Lewin (1950) felt that "hunger pains which are the earliest sequels of rage, are the precursors and prototypes of later self-punishments" (p. 36). I should hasten to add that we would be dealing with *the subjective sensations of* hunger pains. He contrasts these pangs with the narcissistic bliss of satisfaction at the mother's breast. Shame is the subjective, almost reflexive, attempt at self-punishment or self-annihilation accompanying and following the anger at the interruption of narcissistic bliss. The conscious residues and the unconscious memories are illustrated by our child and adult patients who defend themselves from humiliation (and presumed destruction) when they avoid asking us for anything that might be refused. The preconscious fantasy of the expected confrontation followed by sadistic conquest or masochistic submission, murder, or death, is too much to bear. Such patients attempt to control every relationship in or out of the transference that might lead to narcissistic hurt, rejection, or deprivation; for example the patient who always anticipates the end of a treatment session to avoid what is emotionally perceived as the humiliation of forcible abandonment. These reactions are expected most often in patients with pregenital defenses which, of course, include psychosomatic patients.

Depending upon the propensity for defenses against shame and embarrassment, as the individual matures, the affect of shame is closely connected with the loss of more sophisticated personal control. At the time when subjective differentiation from the primary object is in progress, the humiliation, shame, and rage are associated with the subjective experiences of the attempt to control, and the loss of control, over those internal bodily contents, urine and feces. The subjective experience includes the fantasied symbolized internal representations imposed upon the various sensations involved. Specifically, fantasies and feelings associated with internalized object representations and internalized memory traces of events are tied to control and lack of control, to withholding and expulsion. The fantasies are coexistent with the affects of sadistic omnipotence and masochistic shame.

As the child matures and fantasies associated with oral wishes and anal concerns are subjected to their own evolution and maturation, phallic and genital needs take on new significance. Shame becomes associated with sexual submission, possible castration, and desires for sexual penetration. At this point the subject is experiencing phallic and oedipal events, but the same or equivalent affective responses remain to a greater or lesser extent.

What I have so briefly outlined here—an abbreviated development of an important (artificially separated) dynamic affective experience that parallels physiological and behavioral developmental stages—is only a small part of more complex changes in the intermingling affective experiences of the developing individual. In our clinical experience, particularly with narcissistic or psychosomatic patients, we see the defenses against humiliation appear in all these forms. The extent and quality of these appearances depends upon the specific transference regression being experienced or analyzed. With these patients the need for control (or fantasied control) of the environment and of the transference to avoid apparent deprivation, defeat, exposure, and final humiliation, is overwhelming. The defenses we see in the transference of the adult or older child are sophisticated present-day representations of the infantile splitting and denial and its accompanying repression and projective mechanisms.

Herein lies the important dynamic in "alexithymia." The extent of the denial is phenomenal. The projected fantasies of judgment are considered reality by the patient and are unverbalized. Whether or not rage gives rise to McDougall's (1985) idea of the fear of "implosion" or "explosion" would depend upon analyzable content.

In the elaborations of the patient's associations to the transference and life experience, there may be recollections or reconstructions of fantasy life or subjective experience at any level of development. I repeat Lewin's concise explanation: "The unconscious meaning of an event depends on its past history, and the infantile prototype is usually altered by the processes of development" (p. 135).

The content discovered may be visual, verbal, or both. Fantasies with verbal or well-formulated visual content are, in part, derived from later experiences in the patient's development, but more complicated in that such fantasies seem to be part of a telescoping hierarchy of material. A primitive omnipotent anal fantasy of power may be included in a sophisticated idea of nuclear disintegration of planets (the associations to the dream of the patient with masseter spasm cited above).

In patients with psychosomatic disease, a denial of affect may include a denial and repression of content, or a denial and apparently conscious suppression of content. The content may be a split-off fragment or may appear to be consciously suppressed. Here the reason for division is a bit artificial. With conscious suppression the refusal to bring the material into life experience or transference associations is usually rationalized by superego projections. The patient anticipates the pejorative judgments of the analyst or the environment. Even with conscious withholding there is a certain splitting accompanied by projection. The splitting and suppression can be rationalized by innumerable varieties of fantasy: "It is not important," "He (or she) expects me to think this," "I don't really believe this."

Such denial and repression or suppression of content can replicate itself time and time again in successive layers of development. The early affective experience of shame and rage, without words, whatever the content, can set up defenses against the later verbalized experiences of similar shame and rage. The observation that the contemporary fantasy, whether denied or repressed—whether in or out of transference—may seem to evolve from current, recent, or late childhood sources does not in any way separate this material from a succession of more primitive childhood fantasies, which may become available as time and treatment proceed.

On the current transference level, the suppression of fantasies and denial of their importance sometimes gives rise to a state of "alexithymia," in which the fantasy material can become available after what is sometimes a prolonged period of apparently shallow, aimless observations and complaints by the patient. The suppressed fantasies are usually accompanied by projections and projective identifications.

In Freud's traditional concept when pregenital conversion symptoms appear, there is conversion, in time and space, of fantasies involving impulse, pain, and defense, to a physical reaction. Rather there is a physical expression and attempted communication of a simultaneous repressed fantasy, often accompanied by denial, and suppressed conscious fantasies. In patients with psychosomatic problems there are layers of repression and denial accompanied by splitting, fragmentation, projection, and/or projective identification, often provoking countertransference reactions of boredom, inattention, and drowsiness.

Lewin noted (1950, p. 163) that those functions which originally seemed to ward off impulses gradually become substitute gratifications for the things against which they defend. Such an observation is important here, since we find masochistic gratification in the pain of psychosomatic symptoms, as well as a certain elated pleasure in suppressed or expressed sadistic fantasies of omnipotent control. In some patients a conscious scenario of hurt, anger, and complaint, along with pleasurable fantasied controlling sadistic retaliations, accompany the psychoanalytic psychotherapeutic experience for months, but remain unverbalized until the patient experiences the expression of rage as appropriate and justified (the primitive superego gives permission). This expression of righteous indignation is often facilitated by projective mechanisms in the transference. These transference confrontations often give rise to countertransference decisions that the patient is psychotic. It is difficult to respond with analytic precision to an uncontrolled angry outburst (whether unjustified or justified), particularly if it is based on a projection. Yet it is necessary—often without response or interpretation for a duration of days or weeks—if the patient is to become aware of the extent of his own aggression and sadism.

Explosive expressions of affect with subsequent associations, memories, and fantasies are often dramatically therapeutic in that we observe transient or sometimes permanent remission in symptoms (pregenital conversions) with affective release. Such transient remissions in pregenital conversion are likely to become permanent as the simultaneous preconscious and conscious controlling sadistic fantasies (with their erotic elements) are examined and worked through.

I hope to make clear that pregenital conversions are somatic approximations of pregenital fantasies that are simultaneously parallel to the physical symptom, just as the hysterical conversion is a somatic approximation of a simultaneous oedipal fantasy involving phallic and genital wishes and defenses. In both cases the fantasy life is parallel and concurrent with the symptom. One is dealing with parallel data, and the languages that we use to present the data are parallel but different.

As the pregenital conversion (psychosomatic symptom) is given up there is a shift from the physical expression in the organ system (lungs, gut, vascular systems in the dura, etc.) to the more consciously motivated striated muscular activity. Acting out usually occurs as the physical symptom is given up. Subjectively, mildly elated acting out is followed by a psychic shift in which fantasies of victimization and the experience of physical discomfort and pain are replaced with depression and anxiety (often phobic). It reminds me of the Kleinian concept of a shift from the schizoid to the depressive level.

The essential mechanisms of hysterical and pregenital conversions are closely related and the symptom paralleling the subjective conflict seems to depend upon the depth of regression involved. The symptoms do change with the resolution of conflict.

As conflicts are acknowledged and resolved, there is often a shift in pregenital conversions, and one psychosomatic symptom may be replaced with another (Levitan, 1978; Mintz, 1989, see chapter 12, this volume). Migraine headaches or eczema are frequent replacements for episodes of bowel activity in inflammatory colonic disease. These shifts usually, but not always, predate the shift to neurotic disturbances such as depression and anxiety (often phobic) in patients who are undergoing psychoanalytic psychotherapy.

The shift, often with reversals, from pregenital conversions to acting out is close to being a universal progression in successful treatment. As the transference neurosis emerges, the depression and anxiety states become more predictable. However, I have not seen *a progression from a pregenital conversion symptom to a permanent hysterical conversion symptom*, at least not in the area of motor symptoms. If one classifies recurrent simple headaches as a hysterical conversion, these are not infrequent. One should take note of the possible exception, the *transient* symptom of masseter spasm mentioned above.

In brief, pregenital conversion reactions involve those physiological changes not commonly acknowledged to be under conscious control. The parallel and simultaneous fantasies are primitive and deal with pregenital conflicts over aggression, sadism, and humiliation. The primitive nature of their content is accompanied by equally primitive mechanisms of denial, fragmentation, projection, and projective identification.

Chapter 10
The Concept of Stress

Medicine likes its generalities, and stress is a general term. It is certainly too imprecise a concept for the psychoanalytic investigator. Selye (1936, 1950, 1956, 1974) attempted to formulate a unified theory of adaptation and stress, an attempt carrying within it a neglect of particulars.

One can agree with Elliot (1989) when he notes that "The concept that environmental stress can affect health problems probably dates back to the ancients, but the nineteenth century ideal of scientists in pursuit of physical causes for disease tended to minimize the role of agents that could not be seen and quantified" (p. 45). "After 35 years, no one has formulated a completely satisfactory definition of stress, and no ready solution is at hand" (p. 47).

Contemporary ideas of stress and stressors (Selye, 1950) can be traced back to Claude Bernard (1878) and the (again imprecise) regulatory concepts involved in his *milieu interieur*.[1]

Cannon's (1935, 1939) studies on homeostasis and his behavioristic concept of the fight–flight response was an important part of the groundwork for later studies of physiological data on stress in the psychosomatic diseases. He saw stress as a strain on organisms so strong as to push them beyond their adaptive capabilities.

Franz Alexander (1939), Arthur Mirsky (1957), Harold Wolff (1950), Felix Deutsch (1939, 1953), T. P. Almy (1961b),

---

[1]The concept of physiological and psychological regulatory processes within the individual.

and George Engel (1952, 1962), among others, have given us clinical and laboratory evidence of the response of human and animal organisms to outside stimuli, all of which seem to fall under the rubric of stress.

It was Hans Selye (1956) who postulated a nonspecific general adaptation syndrome (GAS) and the more specific local adaptation syndromes (LAS) as well as the highly abstract concept of adaptation energy. His three stages in the GAS syndrome, (1) alarm reaction, (2) stages of resistance, and (3) stage of exhaustion (pp. 58–74) date back to his first publication (1936), "A Syndrome Produced by Certain Nocuous Agents." In 1956 he noted that "in conversation and in lectures I had previously often used the term '*biological stress*' " (p. 30).

Despite Selye's (1950) definitions of stress and stressors, the words themselves have led to a multitude of meanings. The nouns *stress* and *stressors* are totally imprecise. While the latter is commonly utilized to describe a stimulus from the environment, it is also less commonly used to describe internal conflicts. The inexact word *stress* is in common usage as a description of internal bodily tensions, as well as of environmental factors. The adjective-adverb "stressed" lends itself to innumerable uses.

I have already spoken of Mason's (1971) modifications of the general adaptation syndrome (p. 67). I agree with his limitations on the generalities of the syndrome and the specificity of responses. I also agree with his observation that the stress concept should not be regarded primarily as a psychological but rather as a behavioral one. I do find fault with his concept of the independence of mind and brain and his view that mind is a higher order of brain organization.

Koranyi (1989) states that "stress is an elusive concept, a linguistic monster to some, the scrutiny of which poses a considerable methodological challenge to the researcher" (p. 241). Having summed up the concerns of "cellular biologists, immunologists, endocrinologists, and neurophysiologists . . . psychologists and even sociologists" (p. 242) he discusses the simplistic popular use of the term. He notes the confusion when he observes: "Stress is not only biological but can be psychological; is not necessarily adverse but can be challenging and instructive; is not only external but can be internal" (p. 242). Koranyi does a thorough job of summing up the confusion that is involved in defining this extremely ill-defined term, *stress*.

Concepts of stress and of homeostasis have been discussed almost entirely in physiological terms, although a number of authors have attempted to obliterate the duality of data arising from the mind and the body. Some grope for a concept of identity in the idea of stress, but very few recognize that an identity cannot be assumed until one understands the duality in our data with separate linguistic structures, each of which can be representative of that identity.

We may be able to discern such a parallel group of observations if we note that Cannon's (1935) highly abstracted concept of homeostasis may be the physiological counterpart of Freud's equally abstract psychological formulation of the repetition compulsion.

The idea of a psychological constancy coordinating with homeostasis was with Freud all his life. In his "Project" (1895) he discusses it under the name of "neurotic inertia." Despite confusion over points of observation (or sources of data) he alludes to the same thing (1920) when he refers to the psychological need "to keep the quantity of excitation present in it as low as possible, or at least to keep it constant" (p. 9).

I don't think it takes much imagination to see that the processes of homeostasis and regulation in the nervous system, along the hypothalamo-pituitary-adrenocortical axis and other physiological and biochemical systems, is paralleled by Freud's observations of the mind in the abstractions of his metapsychology. We would naturally enjoy more exact one-to-one translations of the coordinates, but these correlations will remain problems for future investigators.

If we want to use stress as a highly abstract noun, which by its nature includes all the particulars of trauma from in the mind and in the mind's perceptions, I guess that it is inevitable.

In both lay literature and the medical press it is constantly utilized in that fashion.

However, it is difficult, since stress and its brother noun *stressor* is also utilized in the same publications, to adequately represent those environmental "nocuous agents" of Selye's (1936). The major part of the experimental literature concerns itself with the observer's environmental provocation of the subject, and recording of the physiological or behavioral response.

One could make a good case for greater accuracy in communication by defining categories of stress: Stress (1) and Stressor (1) for physiological and the environmental, and go on to Stress (2) and Stressor (2) for the psychological and perceptual. And then Stress (3) for the behavioral. The use of such terms might be preferable, but most improbable.

I agree with Koranyi (1989) in considering the abstract noun *stress* a "linguistic monster" (p. 241). I feel that as long as we are going to use it, linguistically it should be confined to physiological and behavioral conceptualizations. There seems to be one certainty. The term has no place in any psychoanalytic linguistic scheme, except perhaps in recognition of its parallel position to disturbance, pain, hurt, or conflict.

But in accordance with popular and medical preference I defer and lodge no further objections. However, I will never mention the word in a psychoanalytic context.

Chapter 11
Alexithymia and Regulatory Processes

ALEXITHYMIA

Alexithymia deserves a heading of its own, even if one feels that the label is misleading and that the category of patients does not represent a valid clinical entity. In recent years it has become such a popular designation and sometimes explanation for certain clinical phenomena that as much as one might like to, one cannot ignore the word.

Pierre Marty, a French psychoanalyst with a great deal of experience in the psychoanalytic investigation of psychosomatic patients (Marty and de M'Uzan, 1963; Marty, de M'Uzan and David, 1963; Marty, 1976; Marty and DeBray, 1989) along with de M'Uzan noted a group of personality characteristics common to many psychosomatic patients. These patients seem to have a dearth of fantasies and their associations were tied to everyday reality and a recitation of activities. Marty and de M'Uzan (1963) gave the name *pensée opératoire* to these character traits. Later Marty and DeBray changed the label to the *vie opératoire*.

Nemiah and Sifneos (1970) noted similar personality characteristics among patients whom they classified as psychosomatic and had seen in investigative interviews. None was in psychoanalysis or psychoanalytic psychotherapy. Then Sifneos (1972, 1973) coined the word *alexithymia* to designate this personality structure.

Since then volumes of literature have arisen around this assumed clinical entity. Much of the early work was included in the volume *Toward a Theory of Psychosomatic Disorders: Alexithymia, Pensée Opératoire, Psychosomatisches Phänomenon* (1977) edited by Bräutigam and von Rad. Then and now attempts have been made to separate psychosomatic from psychoneurotic patients on the basis of this presumed symptom constellation, and it has been noted that alexithymia is present in a number of other pathological conditions not ordinarily thought of as psychosomatic. Numerous descriptions of the symptomatology (Nemiah and Sifneos, 1970; Sifneos, 1972, 1973; Apfel and Sifneos, 1979) as well as tests manufactured to elucidate the presence of alexithymia are found in the literature. Among the earliest and best known of the tests is the *Beth Israel Hospital Psychosomatic Questionnaire* (Sifneos, 1973).

Comments by one of the originators of the concept *pensée opératoire*, Pierre Marty (Marty and DeBray, 1989), may be an appropriate way to initiate our discussion:

> To make a global concept like the *vie opératoire* into an entity, such as the concept of alexithymia seems to have become (the inventors of which have always pointed out that it emerged from *pensée opératoire*), where the emphasis is placed on the impossibility of expressing feelings with words, appears to us unsatisfactory for descriptive and phenomenologic reasons. It is altogether too fixed to recognize the richness and complexity of inter-individual and intra-individual differences throughout the unfolding of a life [p. 182].

Marty and DeBray go on to point out that any person is susceptible to the arrival of what they now call the *vie opératoire* and to possible somatic disorganization. Here the originator of an idea disagrees with the conclusions of his most ardent disciples, Sifneos and Nemiah.

I agree with both of Marty's observations. I've seen massive denial resulting in an apparent lack of fantasy life, lack of dreams, and preoccupation with the mundane facts of everyday life (Hogan, 1983a, p. 120; 1989, pp. 383–385; 1990, p.

229–242). I have presented clinical illustrations of such a defensive posture in inflammatory bowel disease and eating disorders. I have also seen it in patients with migraine headaches, asthma, obsessional disturbances, depression, and other symptoms of psychopathology. I have noted then and now that there is often no clear repression of content but a suppression of affect with a denial of content. Many patients in psychoanalytic psychotherapy or psychoanalysis, once the primitive superego and its precursors can tolerate the denied aggression and sadism, explode in the transference, reciting any and all of the analyst's previous sins, real and imagined, that the patient has observed and fantasied over the preceding months and has been unable to verbalize. These behaviors can be interpreted in a number of ways, but certainly splitting, projection, and projective identification are the main mechanisms involved in the denial. It is apparent that similar attempts at denial are likely to present themselves in other chronic organic illnesses, as so many authors have described (Nemiah, Freyberger, and Sifneos, 1976; Freyberger, 1977).

Some have tried to separate the particular type of denial labeled alexithymia from the defenses utilized in the psychoneuroses (McDougall, 1982b, 1985; Taylor, 1987, p. 84). My own clinical experience has not offered any clear differentiation. In depression and obsessive compulsive conditions one often faces an apparently similar defensive structure. I have noticed such defenses in masochistic patients with a variety of diagnoses.

Wilson (1983b) disagrees with the concept of alexithymia and notes that, "when anorexics and other psychosomatic patients don't report fantasies and dreams, it is a sign of intense resistance that can be analyzed" (p. 245).

Cecil Mushatt (1989) refutes Nemiah and colleagues (Nemiah, Freyberger, and Sifneos, 1976).

According to their proposed theory of alexithymia, patients with psychosomatic disease cannot be treated psychoanalytically, because some inborn defect renders them incapable of fantasy life and appropriate emotional experience. In fact, however, patients with psychosomatic illness are overburdened by primitive emotions and fantasies which their bodily language both defends against and symbolically expresses. This bodily language can be decoded [p. 33].

Knapp (1981) agreed that alexithymia is a defensive process involving massive denial. McDougall, despite her earlier interest in alexithymia (1982a,b, 1985), has distanced herself from the concept (1989):

Analytic observation of these alexithymic and operatory reactions to psychological stress enabled me to see that these were frequently defensive measures against inexpressible pain and fears of a psychotic nature, such as the danger of losing one's sense of identity, of becoming mentally fragmented, perhaps of going mad. To this extent my slowly developing theoretical position differs from the theories of causality advanced by Nemiah and Sifneos, in that they see these as arising largely from neuroanatomical defects [p. 25].

McDougall makes another important observation that agrees with my own investigations reported in this volume and in previous publications (1982a, 1989b). She states (1989):

However, it must be emphasized that many alexithymic and operatory-thinking people do *not* fall somatically ill, and others who suffer from a number of serious psychosomatic maladies do *not* display the operatory and alexithymic character shell that typifies the psychosomatic patients who have been the most studied in psychoanalytic research and in psychosomatic services. On the contrary, in my psychoanalytic practice I have had a number of polysomatizing patients who were intensely aware of their affective experiences [p. 37].

Freyberger (1977), Nemiah, Freyberger, and Sifneos (1976), and Lolas and von Rad (1989), all interested advocates of the concept, make essentially the same observations as

McDougall and myself as we note the ever widening distribution of this assumed diagnostic entity, but they maintain a strong interest in the value and validity of the concept.

McDougall abstracts or generalizes by describing these patients as "disaffected," a term she utilizes to indicate (1989) "a striking absence of affect" (p. 93). I have the same objections here as I have toward the term *alexithymia*. An abstraction can obscure the complexity and richness of defensive maneuvers patients employ to guard against their intense and often chaotic affect and imagery. Generalization tends to transfer the complicated work of decoding (Mushatt, 1989, p. 33) to a pallid label for a process. Second, it is a term for "a striking *absence of affect*" (1989, p. 93) but McDougall agrees in a number of places that there is affect, although not admitted, recognized, or expressed.

I find the concept of alexithymia not only a useless generalization, but also absolutely in error and misleading in its nature. *It places the psychiatrist and patient in a joint conspiracy because both deny the latent subjective mental content that is potentially available.* If psychiatrists, without recognizing their concomitant linguistic error, insist on a neurological, right brain–left brain explanation or some anomalous structural cause, they cannot help the patient verbalize potentially available, but denied, subjective material. Affect and thought may be conscious but suppressed and split off, or it may be temporarily repressed.

I am merely paraphrasing many others. McDougall (1989) refutes Nemiah and Sifneos "in that they see [alexithymia] as arising from neuroanatomical defects . . ." (p. 35). Mushatt (1989) disputes "some inborn defect [that] renders [alexithymics] incapable of fantasy life [or] appropriate emotional experience" (p. 33). We all agree that an emphasis on neuroanatomical defects precludes an investigation of psychic content, the subjective content that certainly parallels the neurological process (see chapter 7).

REGULATORY PROCESSES

A number of contemporary authors have attempted to formulate and organize psychosomatic medicine primarily as a regulatory problem (Schwartz, 1979, 1981, 1983, 1989; Weiner, 1982; Hofer, 1983, 1984; Taylor, 1987; Weiner and Fawzy, 1989; Adler and Adler, 1989). Since so much attention has been directed toward this aspect of psychosomatic medicine, the ideas of regulation and disregulation should be addressed.

Internal regulation of function and attempts to regulate the surrounding environment present problems for any organism. We do not always appreciate that, unlike any other primate, or for that matter any other organism, the human mammal presents us with a unique opportunity. It is the only animal that allows us to examine its organization and the included regulatory processes from two entirely distinct viewpoints. If we use the visual metaphor of a window for each of these fields of observation, we might say that it is our duty to be cognizant of the window that we are looking through. It is also our obligation to be aware of the fact that each window forces upon us use of the appropriate linguistic style for describing the view before us and for recognizing the source of our data.

Over the years we have made some remarkable discoveries about the internal regulatory processes of the human animal, as well as the nature of man's attempts to regulate his environment. In a highly abstracted way, von Bertalanffy (1964, 1968) has clarified for us man's place in the universe with application of his general systems theory. However, the two parallel views of the same phenomena have been obscured in orders of abstraction, and I feel that general systems theory is limited in its application to any strictly defined psychosomatic phenomenon. Von Bertalanffy (1964) acknowledges the dual sources of data in psychosomatic studies, but shoves the problem to one side with the explanatory word *isomorphism*. Despite his earlier admission of duality (his idea perhaps of two entities) he goes on to his general systems theory as though it in some way explained away the dual sources of data in psychosomatic problems.

From the earliest medical observations human beings have shown great interest in how their *milieu interieur* operated anatomically and physiologically. Since the dawn of recorded thought and religion, there has been a similar interest in the organization and regulation of the human mind. In their subjective world, human beings have seen their own minds as encompassing the universe (e.g., some forms of Buddhism), and in most western religions, they have pictured their minds as being totally subservient to the dictates and rules of a greater mind.

It was the physiologist Claude Bernard (1865, 1878) who contributed the first important exposition of the remarkable regulatory physiological processes that the human body automatically performs to keep the *milieu interieur* in an organized, stable condition.

Bernard's work was followed by that of many investigators, both in physiology and psychology. In psychology the most significant ideas were Freud's who expressed early interest in regulatory processes by discussion of constants, neurotic inertia, and repetition compulsion. He also contributed the concept of superego as the abstracted sum of subjective regulatory processes.

A notable high point in research on regulation was achieved by Walter Cannon (1929, 1931, 1935) whose early work on physiological responses that accompany emotional states led to his concept of homeostasis: any organism's physiological as well as emotional stability and organization were essential ingredients in its adaptation to outside stimuli.

F. Deutsch (1922, 1939, 1953, 1959), Franz Alexander (1939, 1950), Daniels (1941), M. Sperling (1949a,b, 1967), Dunbar (1935), Reiser (1975), Weiner (1977), Schwartz (1977, 1979, 1989), Kimball (1981, 1989), Adler and Adler (1989), and Taylor (1987) among many others have contributed to our understanding of regulation and disregulation, both psychologically and physiologically, in psychosomatic disease. A number of these investigators have made generalizations about regulatory mechanisms that include cybernetics, biofeedback, and general

systems theory; others have remained within the more traditional psychoanalytic frameworks. For the most part, confusion
reigns over the sources of data and the languages of transmission of that data: psychological, physiological, or behavioral.
Yet all have taken an interactionist position, which naturally
accompanies a separation of the independent mind versus body
explanation. Even Taylor, who ostensibly agrees with Graham
on the importance of understanding linguistic parallelism, retreats to interactionist understanding of research and clinical
material.

The areas of physiological regulation do concern the psychoanalyst, who looks for simultaneous physiological and behavioral activities to help the patient resolve unconscious subjective conflict. One needs to know the physiology,
pathophysiology, anatomy, pathological anatomy, biochemistry, chemical disregulation, and pharmacology of the psychosomatic disorders one treats. One also needs to know how this
material may parallel subjective states of mind and subjective
conflict, conscious and unconscious. It behooves psychoanalysts
to study epidemiological correlates such as the relationship between bereavement and the onset of disease (Engel and
Schmale, 1967) and to allow ourselves the benefit of generalized
observations evolving from such studies.

With specific reference to regulation, we should know about
the control of the hypothalamo-pituitary-adrenocortical axis
and the important roles played in physiological transmission
and regulation by neuronal transmission and chemical processes. We should also recognize that these studies, for the most
part, describe physiological regulation, and while presumably
its correlation with observations of subjective psychological regulation will become clearer and clearer as time passes, we are
dealing with two separate realms of investigation. The field is
not psychophysiology in any cause-and-effect sense, but a field
of physiological investigation.

For example, the role of corticosteroids in the activity of
the colon is clinically as well as theoretically important to us
both when we utilize them for treatment of inflammation and

when we remove them from a specific therapeutic regimen. We are dealing with physiological regulation. On the other hand, physiological regulation may or may not be of assistance when we deal with evidence of psychological regulation in our setting of psychoanalytic treatment. We are here involved in two different areas of observation: the concept of identity in regulation may be illustrated by simultaneity of observations of data, but causality cannot cross over from one data base to another. Simultaneous mind does not cause physiology (cerebral activity) nor does physiology (cerebral activity) cause simultaneous mind.

Taylor (1987) uses a simple but illustrative research example when he discusses environmental influence on regulation. "The same group studied the effects of friendly dogs on blood pressure and heart rate. They found that touching, talking to, and even simply looking at the animals resulted in lower blood pressure" (p. 291). In this example (as in many "psychosomatic" studies) we are investigating physiological responses to a particular environmental stimulus. We may *assume* accompanying mental (psychological) content when we observe the subjects' behavioral activity and physiological responses. We may see the dog, too, as part of a regulatory process, but this study as reported, is one of environmental regulation of physiology with accompanying behavioral observations.

In an assumption of accompanying mental (psychological) content the psychiatrist could conceivably find that the subject had tender loving feelings toward his or her mental representations of the dog that accompanied the physiological response. The psychoanalyst might, through associations, find the meaning the participant's perceptions of the dog might elicit from the preconscious and the past. But this psychological study would need to accompany the physiological and behavioristic ones. Only then would we have a valid psychosomatic study.

As a matter of fact, the study might be more revealing (and scientific) than the simple tyranny of a statistical majority. One could guess that in any given series there might be at least one subject who had internalized, for whatever reason, a hostile mental representation of our canine friends, contributing to an elevation in blood pressure. Statistics do not contribute much to individual psychological understanding. Here we need individual studies of subjective content, not a statistical majority of physiological or behavioral responses.

When treating psychosomatic diseases psychoanalytically, we are continuously aware of the psychological representations of regulatory processes as we observe the activity of the superego and its precursors. (In primitive regressions we sometimes characterize the activity of this regulatory superego as sadistic because of the shame, humiliation, and masochistic wishes experienced by the ego in response to the demands of a primitive self-directing organization.) In the patient who utilizes pregenital defenses extensively (true of psychosomatic patients), the early subject and object representations are internalized primitive perceptions of part self and part objects from an archaic level of development, introjects which constitute an inadequately organized part of the subjective regulatory apparatus, the superego. However, in treatment, both patient and psychoanalyst can discern and eventually understand specific conflicts between specific fragments (internalized representations of part objects) and specific impulses with their accompanying fantasies.

In the psychoanalytic process we do not intend to end up with generalizations. We expect to understand specific conflicts from the past that still exist in the mind of the patient usually represented by contemporary conflict.

The subjective representation of a controlling agency in the mind may be accompanied by simultaneous self-destructive physical responses such as asthma or inflammatory bowel disease; or self-destructive behavioral disturbances such as masochistic acting out. We can trace the current correlate physiological and psychological disregulations to simultaneous infantile disregulations if we follow our nonmanipulative psychoanalytic principles.

Such material may become available because, in the patient's subjective world, he is able to use a transference object, the analyst, to represent and understand unconscious conflict with perceptions of earlier perceived regulators from environment. These internalized conflicts are primarily derived from perceived conflicts with parents, siblings, and surrogates—*subjectively* experienced as our patient relates to current objects (people) in the environment. We can abstract the regulatory aspects of these particulars under the generalizations of superego and superego precursors.

All of these perceptions are accompanied by content and affect. Experiences with current objects, whether in the transference with the psychoanalyst or other important people, give rise to current fantasy and affect. As a psychoanalyst one works with the meaning of this content for the patient, and the patient often recalls past experiences and conflicts antedating and conditioning current subjective experiences. When an investigator is interested only in a subject's behavioral response to an objectively (clearly the investigator's subjectively) observed and evaluated stimulus the investigator is involved in a behavioral and not a psychological study of the individual.

From a behavioristic and physiological point of view we may see external events and stimuli as regulators, as in the case of the blood pressure and the pups above. Here we have a behavioristic statistical tabulation of physiological responses to our environmental stimuli, which in aggregate we may see as regulators. These regulators are environmental and give rise to physiological or behavioral data. The investigator may assume an understanding of the subjective experiences of the participant, but has no evidence that one has more than a tabulation of experiences of a statistical majority of participants.

Taylor's (1967) examples of regulation and deregulation covered an immense amount of experimental and clinical material, which he fitted into Kohut's developmental theory of self–object relationships (and regulations). Taylor's discussion of this concept and its justification from clinical material as opposed to the more traditional drive–conflict theories in psychoanalysis are too elaborate and too profound an argument to approach in this volume. I do differ, however, with his views on regulation and one's approach to the patient. Any study must, I feel, include an accurate description of our frames of observation—are these subjective and psychological with linguistic communication, or are we observing behavioral responses of the subject (patient) to outside physical environmental effects?

Taylor and many other investigators (psychologists, psychiatrists, and psychoanalytic psychiatrists of diverse schools of thought) are inclined to lump such spheres of observation together as equivalents. In chapters 9 and 10 (1987), Taylor makes observations of parallel or unrelated events and assumes a causal intermix without seeming recognition or presentation of the multitudinous frames of reference.

One could, I suppose, think of apples and oranges. He feels, perhaps correctly, that a number of things assist the patient in the control of his behavior, physiology and subjective mental experience. These "regulators" seem to include environmental items such as social relationships, pets, placebos, and doctors. (I realize I do an injustice to the variety and depth of the research material in such a brief summary, but I have an important academic point to make.) Taylor's commingling of subjective states, behaviors, relationships and objects, in my opinion, calls most of his conclusions into question. I am more confused when he equates stimuli with the *self–object of primary identification* (p. 301). I agree that the example he cited, the "reclining chair," that he assumed was a regulating presence, may have had subjective meaning to the patient, if we add that the perception of that chair may call subjective internal associations, internalizations, and memories into the preconscious and conscious realms of affective and ideational experience. But his example is absolutely not psychology. There is no subjective material presented relating the reclining chair to the patient's internal world of affect, meaning, or conflict. The chair is a chair, is a chair. It is not by itself a self–object of primary identification.

We must remember that in the realm of object relations we are dealing with the patient's fantasied elaborations of perceptions of the real "object of primary identification" (p. 301). It

is true that the patient utilizes such all inclusive object representations (internalizations of primitive part objects in more traditional language) for perceived self-regulation or perceived environmental regulation. We are only justified in using object
relations theory in the psychoanalytic situation when we deal
with the subjective associations of, and meanings to, the patient.
We are not justified in arbitrarily inferring that a pet, placebo,
chair, or piece of social support is, by our saying so, taking
any particular object's place, unless the patient's associations
indicate that subjective meaning.

True, in eclectic psychotherapy we use social support, physician's reassurance, placebos, and other external manipulations
to provide quick and effective aid and they have a demonstrable
value in the amelioration of symptoms in many instances. However, eclectic psychotherapy is not psychoanalysis, nor does it
discriminate among various platforms of observation. It is not
a research tool. We may at times infer subjective meaning to
pieces of changed behavior, and I should not object if we related this behavior to an environmental object such as a chair
so long as one is clear that it is only an inference. However,
Taylor (1967, p. 301) jumps over to the field of object relations;
his connection of that chair via Grotstein (1981, 1983) to Winnicott's (1965) environmental mother is a questionable exercise.

There is little doubt about the importance of regulation and
disregulation as one of many physiological and psychological
abstractions. But it is critical that we recognize which frame of
observation or linguistic mode we use to support our observations. The authors displaying an interest in the relevance of a
psychosomatic explanation or doctrinal formulation (Weiner,
1982; Taylor, 1987; Schwartz, 1989) take interactionist positions. To allow crossovers of subjective data with implied envi-
ronmentally or physiologically induced physiological or behavioral states is a crucial semantic error, particularly true when
the author (Taylor, 1987) recognizes and accepts empirically
demonstrable linguistic parallelism.

Self-regulation and attempts at environmental regulatory
manipulation are only aspects of the complex physiological,

neurophysiological and biochemical processes that we observe and describe in the sphere of physical observation. In the parallel sphere of psychic activity, subjective self-regulation and subjective attempts at subjectively perceived environmental regulation are also only aspects of dynamic psychic processes. In the language of psychoanalysis, most regulatory processes fall in the area of those abstractions of subjective processes, the superego and its precursors.

The oversimplification and reduction of all the complexities of object relations as seen and interpreted in the psychoanalysis of a psychosomatic patient to the object as a regulator and the doctor as a regulatory object, ignores the vicissitudes of transference and the use of transference to relive and find solutions to past conflicts (Otto Sperling [1980] cited by Taylor [1987, p. 307]).

The field of psychosomatic medicine has far greater depth and dimension than psychological regulation and disregulation. I believe that treatment requires a more discrete recognition of the minute areas of psychological conflict that may be distantly related but far removed from material involving subjective regulation. There is more to the content of body and to the content of subjective experience (mind) than *milieu interieur*. *Milieu interieur* is a very high order of abstraction and cannot be placed on the same level as physiological and psychological mechanisms, whether in the language of body or the language of mind. When we speak of *milieu interieur* (1) body, we use a different order of observation than we do when speaking of *milieu interieur* (2) mind. Among these discrete psychological observations, the state of the transference is of utmost importance and requires more sophisticated understanding of emotion, fantasy, and memory than simply "doctor as object." At the same time both patient and physician should recognize simultaneous observations of physiology, behavior, and body in the parallel linguistic areas. There is no spatial *interface* (Taylor, 1987, p. 172) between the "psychological" and the "neurobiological."

At this point in the review of concepts of regulation and disregulation we can broaden our outlook to include physiological and behavioral approaches of psychiatrists to the field of psychosomatic medicine. Lawrence Deutsch (1980) offered an informed summary and some interesting observations on work reviewed in four volumes devoted to psychosomatic medicine (Lipowski, Lipsitt, and Whybrow, 1977; Usdin, Hamburg, and Barchas, 1977; Weiner, 1977; Wittkower and Warnes, 1977).

Most of the material reviewed dealt primarily with physical, physiological, social, and epidemiological studies. L. Deutsch (1980) noted that "life experiences in the studies cited measure events, not affects. Affective responses to events should also be correlated with disease and represent an intervening variable" (p. 666). L. Deutsch's emphasis on the subjective, the affect, is undoubtedly correct, but he presents affect as an intervening variable in a chain of linear causality, rather than relating the parallel nature of affect (one of mind's functions) to the physical events.

Unfortunately, he observed that he did not find "more than a limited role for psychoanalytic doctrine or approaches in psychosomatic medicine . . ." (p. 684).

After a discussion of the physiological data, Deutsch reminds the reader of Freud, Groddeck, Fenichel, F. Deutsch, Schilder, Schur, M. Sperling, Federn, Hartmann, Mushatt, and Wilson. He discusses therapeutic successes associated with psychoanalysis and psychoanalytic psychotherapy and notes: "Frequently, after successful interpretation and working through of psychosomatic symptoms, neurotic symptoms (phobias, depression), psychotic symptoms, acting out or accident proneness replace physiological manifestations" (p. 696). His views accord nicely with the observations in this volume. I fully concur with Deutsch's conclusion that "psychoanalysis can serve as a primary research tool and therapeutic modality in the field of psychosomatic medicine" (p. 699).

At issue is the attempt to broadly generalize and abstract models, usually based primarily on physical and behavioral

data. These generalizations, whether in the sphere of physiological regulation and disregulation, or even in the parallel data
base of psychological regulation and disregulation, are unjusti-
fiably limiting concepts. To proceed to mix the two areas of
observation, the mind and the physical, in an interactionist
manner is not only an oversimplification, it is a downright error.

I agree with L. Deutsch (1980) that we are dealing with
complex groups of observations from a variety of areas of observation. It is of obvious value to use concepts of regulatory
mechanisms and disregulation when we evaluate our data from
the area of physical observation. It is also of value to group our
data in regulatory terms (such as superego) when we examine
findings from the parallel area of psychological experience.
When our parallel languages achieve the necessary accuracy,
as the translations of simultaneous records in our dictionaries
are honed further, our knowledge takes on a new dimension.
Now we can often conclude an identity. Whether we wish to
use this information in a regulatory or in a broader context will
depend on the immediate purpose of our communication.

In evaluating subjective data we cannot help but pay our
respects to the general outline of psychoanalytic thought. In its
concept of drive–defense conflict, psychoanalysis has provided
the physician with the tool that has led most consistently to
therapeutic success in the psychological treatment of psychosomatic symptoms. In our psychoanalytic studies we note the patients' physical observations of themselves as well as medical
evaluations by our associates. Psychoanalysis as a research tool,
as an in-depth study of the organization of the personal psyche,
has contributed more than any other method of investigation
to our understanding of the psychopathology of psychosomatic
illnesses.

True, there have been new discoveries with consequent re-
formulations of theoretical positions (most notably in the areas
of early development and pregenital defenses). There have
been corollary modifications in therapeutic activity (primarily
in more active early interpretation of defenses). Nevertheless,

the traditional psychoanalytic stance remains that of a neutral, noninterfering, minimally participating observer offering interpretations of subjective conflict, which the patient can experience and evaluate in the context of life's long evolution.

Part III
Psychoanalytic Treatment

Chapter 12
Clinical Review

As we approach the specific application of psychoanalytic principles to the treatment of inflammatory processes in the gut, it is imperative that any participating physician recognize the potential difficulties and complications inherent in handling these illnesses. There have been innumerable cautionary tales from medical and surgical specialists warning of the serious nature of these disease processes; at times recommendations are accompanied by absolute interdictions of any psychoanalytic treatment. Many psychoanalysts feel that such prohibitions are more than open to question, particularly when one compares the long-term results of pharmaceutical supportive therapy with the results of careful psychoanalytic psychotherapy.

As I noted in 1989, "Patients with inflammatory bowel disease present special problems. If handled poorly, their illness can rapidly prove fatal" (p. 381). M. Sperling (1955a, 1957, 1968), among many others, noted potential difficulties and complications and contributed specific recommendations.

I offer my own comments about possible difficulties as Part III unfolds, but I should also make clear that experience has demonstrated that an interested psychoanalytic physician can handle these patients with safety, and in a large number of cases, achieve gratifying results.

I return once again to Otto Sperling's (1978a) observation that there have been many important contributions by psychoanalytic investigators to the field of psychosomatic medicine. He implied that many were more inclined to work with broad samples in the fields of theory and clinical speculation than to get involved in careful day-to-day investigation utilizing psycho-analysis and psychoanalytic psychotherapy: "not many psycho-analysts are willing to take on a psychosomatic case for treat-ment" (p. 6).

I hope that we psychosomatic clinicians can arouse the inter-est of a greater number of psychoanalytic physicians in the intensive treatment of psychosomatic conditions such as the inflammatory diseases of the large bowel.

CLINICAL EXPERIENCE

At this point we begin a review of clinicians who have had an interest in the psychodynamic features of patients with in-flammatory diseases of the gut. Among them are some who have utilized psychoanalytic and/or psychoanalytic psychother-apeutic modalities in the treatment of these patients.

It seems appropriate to begin this chapter with Weinstock's (1962) summary of the work of psychoanalysts and the outcome of their treatment of ulcerative colitis. I go into some detail here because studies of psychoanalytic outcomes, such as Wein-stock's, have been rare. The concentrated nature of psychoana-lytic treatment, three to five times per week, and the extended treatment time precludes the possibility of frequent publication of large series of cases. In this sense Weinstock's report is of unusual significance.

> In order to evaluate the effect of adequate treatment of this disease by experienced psychoanalysts in this country, a national survey was carried out during the past 2 years. To allow not only for treatment but for at least 3 years' follow-up observation after completion of treatment, only members of the American Psychoanalytic Association of at least 5 years' standing were in-vited to participate in this survey. Of the 600 5-year-or-more members, 400 indicated their interest, and of these there were 45 analysts who had treated or were treating a total of 68 cases of ulcerative colitis.

Excluded from this report are:

(1) 12 cases that had inadequate treatment, i.e. from a few months to a year.

(2) 15 cases that are still in treatment.

(3) 4 cases that had previous intestinal operations.

(4) 4 cases that were not severe enough ever to have required hospitalization. These were considered at this time to fall into the mild form of the disease.

(5) 3 cases in which the follow-up is only of 2 years' duration at this time.

(6) 2 cases that were immediately lost to follow-up.

A further report on these cases will be made in proper time.

Thus, this report is limited to 28 cases reported by 20 analysts. All of these cases fulfill the following conditions:

(1) They were cases of severe ulcerative colitis that had required previous hospitalization.

(2) They sought treatment from psychoanalysts for their ulcerative colitis, i.e. in the hope that such treatment would prevent recurrences.

(3) They had periods of psychotherapy or psychoanalysis for a minimum of 2 years (with the exception of 5 cases, whose treatment lasted about 1½ years each).

(4) All of these cases were followed for at least 3 years, most of them for much more than 3 years.

Of the 28 cases, 14 were in psychotherapy, ranging from 1–4 times a week and extending from 1½ years (in 2 cases) to 5 years; and 14 were in analysis averaging 4 times per week and lasting from 1½ years (in three cases) to 5 years.

Of the 14 cases that were in psychotherapy, 12 were totally symptom-free 3–18 years after conclusion of treatment. Of these 12 cases, 2 have had remissions of 3 years so far. The other 10 have remissions of 7–18 years, the median of all being 10 years. In 10 of these 12 cases, the analyst was of the opinion that treatment was carried on as long as he thought necessary.

In the 2 cases in which results were not good, the treatment was not considered adequate in duration by the analyst. In 1 of these 2 cases, frequent recurrences were present during the 2 years of treatment, as they had been for 6 years before, and the patient discontinued treatment against advice. In the other case, after 1½ years of treatment, the patient moved to another city and had a symptom-free period of 5 years, then a short recurrence, followed by 2 years of remission so far. This patient had had unremitting chronic ulcerative colitis for 13 years, experiencing relief for the first time after half a year of treatment.

The group of 14 cases that had extensive periods of analysis showed approximately similar results. Ten of the 14 have had excellent follow-up records of long remissions. Of these 10 good results, 1 case has had a remission of 3 years so far. The other 9 range from 5 to 16 years of symptom-free remission, the median of all being 8½ years. (It must be borne in mind that the treatment of all cases in this survey terminated at various times in the past. Only after the passage of an equal number of years of follow-up on each case may one establish a true average. The median, therefore, is used instead.)

In 8 of these 10 cases, the analytic treatment had been considered complete. In 2 cases treatment was not considered sufficient by the analyst, extending, in one instance for 1½ years with an 11-year remission and, in the other instance, lasting for 3 years with a 6-year remission.

Of the 4 cases that did not do well, 1 was unimproved after 5 years of treatment, 1 had a severe recurrence after 5 years of analysis, 1 had severe recurrences during treatment and in the 3 years of follow-up, and 1 case had a rapidly fatal outcome during analytic treatment for a moderately severe recurrence. . . .

Lest there be doubt about the severity of this group of cases, in each instance the fact of severity was verified through additional communication with the analyst and/or the patient's physician, and the severe symptoms—high fever, large weight loss, skin disorders, joint disturbances, hemorrhages, severe diarrhea—all were corroborated. Of these 28 cases, 5 were hospitalized 1 time only. The rest required from 2 to 13 periods of hospitalization. Leaving out the 1 instance of 13 hospitalizations, the average of all the rest was close to 3 hospitalizations . . . [pp. 244–245].

Interesting, too, is the fact that the successful results were unrelated to the psychiatric diagnoses or the choice of psychotherapy or psychoanalysis as treatment. . . . *Thus, this survey suggests that adequate treatment by psychoanalysts offers a greater possibility for long-term remissions, or perhaps cure, in the severe remitting type of ulcerative colitis than any other treatment, with the exception of surgery* [p. 248, emphasis added].

Before reviewing the work of other clinicians, we must return to the original observer of the role of the mind in the activities of the colon. His notable contributions have been mentioned earlier. Cecil D. Murray[1] (1930a,b), while working as a medical student at George Draper's Constitution Clinic, College of Physicians and Surgeons, Columbia University, was the first person to recognize and document the psychological concomitants to the physical changes in ulcerative colitis.

In his first paper (1930a) Murray discussed:

[An] investigation into the life histories and mental attitudes of 12 patients suffering from bloody diarrhea or ulcerative colitis [which] revealed a close association between the emergence of a difficult psychological situation and the onset of symptoms. . . . In each case the patients faced their problems in an infantile manner [p. 248].

In his second paper (1930b) he referred to the 12 patients but went into detail in his discussion of the "psychological analysis" of a 29-year-old female patient. He noted (pp. 617–618) that although this patient was described as "nervous" she did not complain of mental symptoms and would not have fallen into the group ordinarily referred to the psychiatric clinic. He felt that these patients were inclined to depreciate psychic pain and did not fall into any traditional diagnostic category (pp. 617–618).

---

[1] I should like to note Murray's quite distinguished, but unfortunately short, academic career. He received his A.B. degree from Harvard in 1919 and his Ph.D. from Cambridge in 1925 before entering Columbia University's College of Physicians and Surgeons in 1928. After his work and research as a medical student, he interned at and joined the staff of New York Hospital. On July 4, 1935, at the age of 37 he suffered an untimely death from Hodgkin's disease. We can only speculate as to what further contributions this insightful young physician might have made in his chosen field of physiology if he had had more time. (This biographical information was generously made available by F. R. Hunter, Senior Research Assistant, Division of Library and Information Management of The American Medical Association.)

When patients with inflammatory gut disease first enter treatment, there is a lack of clear definition in traditional psychiatric diagnosis. My own work indicates (1989) that I had "as yet made little mention of traditional psychiatric diagnosis . . . [no patients] at the time of consultation fell into any readily definable, traditional diagnostic category" (pp. 376–377). I referred to Giovacchini's (1977) comment that "the defensive constellation of my patient was vital to maintaining a total ego coherence instead of dealing with discrete conflicting disruptive impulses" (p. 10).

Murray indicated that his patient presented a helpless masochistic temperament that covered suppressed and repressed aggression (sadism). He reported (1930b) that:

> this mechanism [the oedipal interpretation] is overshadowed. . . . Her character and her sexuality corresponded quite closely to the so-called anal level described by Freud and the masochistic and sadistic components . . . were very conspicuous in this patient. . . . The patient's masochism was more in evidence than her sadism . . . her sadism was beneath the surface and manifested itself mostly in neurotic ways [p. 623].

When one reviews his case history, one cannot help but be impressed by the violent sadistic and masochistic fantasy and dream life of this young woman. Cannibalistic content was common. The repressed and denied sadism and masochism in such apparently passive and accommodating people is addressed in chapter 13.

A. J. Sullivan and his colleague at Yale–New Haven Hospital (Sullivan and Chandler, 1932) became interested in Murray's work and reported on six cases, noting that "the patients have been helped more by procedures directed toward the improvement of their personal problems than by medical therapy directed toward the colon" (p. 795).

In 1935 Sullivan reviewed 15 cases ranging from "the acute fulminating type of one month's duration" to the "more usual one of 6 or 7 years duration with numerous remissions and recurrences" (p. 65). He discovered that "they showed few outward signs of bottled up emotion. They seemed to suppress the usual methods of expressing anger, despair, triumph, and were often considered to be rather nonchalant by their friends. . . . Rarely, if ever, is the fundamental problem discussed by the patient at the first or second interview" (p. 652).

Here Sullivan described a state of denial which was later categorized and unfortunately labeled "alexithymia" (Sifneos, 1972, 1973; Nemiah and Sifneos, 1970). He added (1935): "In many cases the specific psychological episodes were related by the patient only after long and persistent questioning" and that "Psychotherapy in most of these cases produced striking results when many other forms of therapy had failed" (p. 655).

Sullivan (1935) also described the intense attachment these patients have to a mother or a surrogate. He emphasized their "helplessness" and "giving up." He observed that colitis patients are "to a large extent of a rather egoistic or narcissistic type. . . . They would withstand rather poorly emotional deprivations" (p. 652).

Unfortunately, none of the reported cases was seen in psychoanalytic psychotherapy. Sullivan felt, however, that his observation confirmed Murray's findings.

During this same period G. E. Daniels had been working with ulcerative colitis patients (1941, 1942). He first reported on this material in his discussion of Sullivan's (1935) paper and said that he had been working with 12 cases over the previous year. He specifically agreed with Sullivan, but later added (1941): "many cases of ulcerative colitis show clear-cut relationships to emotional difficulties, and, in many instances improvement of the condition goes hand in hand with the resolution of the conflict" (p. 1731).

Shortly after this (1942) he discusses his study of 25 cases over ten years, and in referring to Alexander's comparison of the colonic type of personality to the compulsive neurotic, Daniels pointed out:

My impression is that the difference lies in the more narcissistic organization of the personalities in ulcerative colitis, with the

underlying reaction being more a psychotic than a psychoneurotic one. In some cases the symptoms mask a severe depression. . . . In several cases, the disease seemed definitely a type of
organic suicide . . . there is a direct relation between the severity
of the physical reaction and the underlying psychopathology [p.
183].

During this same period in the early 1930s van der Heide of
Holland was doing unpublished work. J. Groen (1947) reported
that in 1938 at the Wilhelmina Gasthaus of Amsterdam, van
der Heide had demonstrated the presence of emotional disturbances in all of the ulcerative colitis patients in the hospital.
Groen concluded that "He [van der Heide] fully confirmed
Murray's findings" (p. 155).

Groen and his coworkers (Groen, 1947, 1951; Groen and
Bastiaans, 1954; Groen and Van der Valk, 1956; Groen and
Birnbaum, 1968) were involved in studies of inflammatory
bowel disease, and all were impressed by the sense of humiliation that accompanied the perceived loss of the object. In general their emphasis was on supportive therapy. In his 1956
paper with Van der Valk there was the repetition: "It is a striking fact, however, that of all those who have tried to repeat
Murray's work there is none, so far as we are aware, who has
failed to confirm fundamental observation" (p. 572).

Lindemann (1945, 1950) had also been working with ulcerative colitis since the 1930s. He (1945) called attention to the
importance of "various forms of bereavement as the most important precipitating factor" and to the paucity of emotional
relationships:

The personality of the patient was marked by poverty of human
relationships, an inability to make and hold friends of their own
age and by a need for considerable activity throughout the day
but lack of resourcefulness in finding avenues for such activity
[p. 322].

Lindemann (1945) also called attention to the overwhelming
anxiety experienced by ulcerative colitis patients, a fear of being

overcome by their primitive impulses. Unfortunately, he cautioned physicians to avoid psychoanalytic psychotherapy, but recommended psychological management. "The technique of psychologic management must avoid the traditional methods of psychoanalytic inquiry . . . not permitting the development of regressive tendencies, hostile feelings or affectionate attachment. The relationship must, rather, be an identifying one" (p. 322). In general Lindemann is notable for his initiation of replacement therapy and the supportive treatment of ulcerative colitis.

Prugh (1950, 1951), Department of Pediatrics, Harvard Medical School, observed and carried out experimental studies on a series of 12 patients during the 1940s. He observed (1951) that with the "appearance of spontaneous or experimentally induced angry or aggressive emotions [there was] . . . an immediate activation of a hypermotile colonic response" (pp. 353–354).

He had noted: "It appears clearly established that an emotional component was active in all of the 12 cases seen in the series" (p. 352). He further observed that they were "children with dependent rigid immature personalities" (p. 353).

Prugh also agreed with the earlier observations of Murray and his followers, Daniels, Sullivan, Sperling, van der Heide, Groen, and Lindemann that these children (as well as adults) maintained a dependent, helpless attachment to their mothers, surrogates, or their internalized representations.

Melitta Sperling (1946) was one of the early investigators who felt that psychoanalysis or psychoanalytic psychotherapy was the treatment of choice. She had begun the psychoanalysis of children with ulcerative colitis in 1942. In 1946 she reported on the treatment of eight children. In 1957, when she reported on the treatment of an adult with ulcerative colitis, she also noted that the original eight were still well. In 1969 she stated: "from 1942 to the present I have treated twenty-one patients intensively and eleven for shorter periods of time" (p. 348). In the same paper she observed: "somatic symptoms are meaningful and are [a] (preverbal) way of expressing and discharging

feelings and conflicts of which [one] . . . is not aware consciously" (p. 349). She recommended "the emphasis in treatment is to encourage the patient to wean himself from medications and medical treatment. This approach is dramatically
different from the team approach" (p. 349). She asserted that
"Ulcerative colitis is not a disease of adulthood as is commonly
assumed. It originates in childhood, although it may remain
latent and the clinical manifestations may appear only later in
life . . ." (p. 338). "The disposition to react with bodily symptoms to emotional trauma is acquired very early in life. In fact
in infants and very young children bodily pathways are the only
outlets for distress arising from any source" (p. 339).

Sperling has often been criticized for her insistence that
somatic symptoms represented unconscious symbols and fantasies. For example (1978a), she noted the increase in symptomatic recurrences when children were placed in hospitals:

> It disrupted their narcissistic equilibrium . . . To the child it
> meant the loss of the mother and being helplessly left to destruc-
> tion, a fate which could be avoided only by setting into motion
> the archaic mechanism of oral sadistic incorporation of the
> needed object with all the destructive somatic consequences of
> the defense mechanism . . . these children are in a state of per-
> manent frustration that results in a state of unconscious rage
> with an irresistible urge for immediate discharge. . . . The de-
> struction and elimination of the object through the mucosa of
> the colon (bleeding) would seem to be the specific mechanism
> in ulcerative colitis. . . . As the object is incorporated sadistically,
> it is a hostile inner danger and has to be eliminated immediately.
> The feces and blood (in severe attacks, only blood and mucus)
> represent the devaluated and dangerous objects [p. 97].

In numerous other writings Sperling illustrates clinical material with specific fantasies, symbols, and symbolic actions.

She explains that "ulcerative colitis is an organ neurosis with
pregenital conversion symptoms. The anorexia, vomiting, abdominal pain, diarrhea, and bleeding represent expressions of

and defenses against aggressive incorporation of the frustrating object" (p. 98).

She (1963) sees the subjectively experienced impulses and unconscious or conscious fantasy life as causative in the production of physiological changes. With the introduction of linguistic parallelism and the recognition that parallel sets of data are involved (see chapters 6 and 7), this fantasy material would be characterized differently. Nevertheless, Sperling's observations have been corroborated by me (see chapter 13) as well as by other psychoanalysts. (I feel that some of the greatest critics of the importance of symbolization and fantasy are often psychoanalytic theorists who have had little direct experience in the psychoanalytic therapy of psychosomatic patients.)

Melitta Sperling has presented impressive clinical material. I should inform the reader that some of my colleagues and I, who are members of the Psychosomatic Discussion Group of the Psychoanalytic Association of New York, Inc., have seen some of Sperling's cases in follow-ups for various reasons and the results remain impressive.

As early as 1969 she reported: "I have follow-up studies from three to twenty-three years on the patients whom I have treated for ulcerative colitis" (p. 348). She also noted: "I was able to achieve a complete cure with a follow-up from five to fourteen years in five children aged three to five years. I have seen similar results in supervision of the treatment of young children with ulcerative colitis" (p. 350). In 1964 she published a twenty-year follow-up study on a child whom she had successfully treated for severe ulcerative colitis when he was 7½ years old.

I have yet to see comparable results in any series of pharmaceutically treated patients—even any group of patients from presteroid days. In many studies from that earlier period patients seemed to have greater life expectancies and fewer complications than do our current crop (Karush, Daniels, Flood, and O'Connor, 1977).

Another among the psychoanalytic pioneers, D. Jackson (1946), made a notable contribution to psychoanalytic understanding of ulcerative colitis when he reported on a case successfully treated with psychoanalysis.

Cushing (1953) presented the successful psychoanalytic treatment of a man suffering from ulcerative colitis. Cecil Mushatt (1954), in an excellent paper, described his experience with eight adult cases of ulcerative colitis, all of whom were seen over a long period of time. He utilized as an example the treatment of a 15½-year-old male treated with psychoanalytic psychotherapy. A notable occurrence in the treatment was the patient's regression into a psychotic episode before progressing to an ultimate remission. Subsequently, Mushatt (1975, 1989; personal communications) has described successful treatment with other cases.

H. Sidney Klein (1965) reported on six cases studied, two of whom were psychoanalyzed. One of the latter developed a clinical psychosis in the transference and the other showed megalomanic features that were confined to the analytic situation. Despite the severe temporary regressions both recoveries were evidently satisfactory.

Robert Savitt (1977) reported a man who came into psychoanalysis as a final step to avoid colectomy. He was in psychoanalytic treatment for four years and terminated treatment after a complete remission. His physical health remained good twenty-five years later. Savitt indicated in a personal communication that he has successfully treated other cases.

Lefebvre (1988) reported on a case utilized as a taking-off point for theoretical discussion. The patient's emotional state was evidently improved but his physical condition would be hard to evaluate because a colectomy was performed for polyps in the midst of the analysis.

M. Aisenstein (1993) reported on a case of haemorrhagic rectocolitis that she had treated in psychoanalytically oriented psychotherapy on a one-session-per-week schedule with notable success.

I propose to forego any further individual case histories from the literature, and proceed to present some clinical material most generously supplied by two of my colleagues, C. Philip Wilson and Ira L. Mintz, in personal communications. The material is quoted as it was presented in letter form. The only exceptions are my parenthesized deletions.

The following is clinical material presented by C. Philip Wilson (1989, personal communication):

My experience with ulcerative colitis:

Case 1. A 25-year-old married woman with chronic ulcerative colitis. When colitis cleared in analysis, she had migraine which was then resolved: ten years analysis, four times a week. Successful resolution of her personality disorder. The case is described on pp. 27–28 of our psychosomatic book (Wilson and Mintz, 1989), describing psychosomatic symptoms replaced by perversions. Diagnosis: Neurotic.

Case 2. Described on p. 117 of our book (Wilson and Mintz, 1989) (identificatory material deleted) ulcerative colitis (28-year-old woman). She resolved her colitis and personality disorder in eleven years of analysis, four times a week. She had a transference psychosis (p. 117). Diagnosis: Borderline.

There are ten-year follow-ups on both cases showing successful results.

Case 3. A 14-year-old boy was seen for a year's analysis, three times a week, with symptom resolution and characterologic change. No follow up, although the parents agreed to bring him back if more symptoms developed. Diagnosis: Neurotic.

Case 4. (whom you [Hogan] referred). A 23-year-old man with severe ulcerative colitis is described on pp. 109–110 (Wilson and Mintz, 1989). He had an excellent result, symptom resolution, and characterological change. His colitis, however, was replaced by anorexia nervosa (Wilson and Mintz, 1989, pp. 69–70). Diagnosis: Neurotic.

Case 5. was a 30-year-old married woman with ulcerative colitis as an adolescent who was analyzed by M. Sperling. She evidenced no further colitis (ten-year follow-up) but came for the analysis of conflicts about getting pregnant, which she resolved, with the result that she had a healthy baby. She had further conflicts, however, and was referred to another psycho-analyst who analyzed her further. Diagnosis: Neurotic.

As you know, I have been analyzing the mother of your [Hogan's] Crohn's disease patient (identificatory material de-leted). The mother is an anal character and her gut crackles on the couch, which has been analyzed. Diagnosis: Borderline.

Those supervised: the treatment of ten other cases of ulcera-tive colitis with effective results, all analytic psychotherapy.

Those analyzed: two cases of spastic colitis, one case of a psychically caused anal wound. One case of regional ileitis [Crohn's ileitis] who acted out after a year and went to surgery, which removed the symptom. She did not return for further therapy.

The following is clinical material presented by Ira L. Mintz (1990, personal communication):

1. Karla, a 24-year-old teacher, entered three times a week analytic psychotherapy with a ten-year history of severe ulcera-tive colitis with approximately thirty-five bloody diarrhea stools a day, cramps, mucus, fever, and generalized malaise. After two-and-one-half years of therapy, the bloody stools were reduced to two a day, along with concomitant reduction of other associated symptoms. Her general health, relationships with people, and professional life satisfactions had all improved markedly.

Prior to beginning treatment, she had been sigmoidoscoped almost weekly for a number of years. When another physician informed her that it was unnecessary, she became enraged, felt exploited, and refused further observation and medical treat-ment, in spite of my pointing out its importance. One day she reported an abdominal mass. Surgical exploration revealed three primary carcinomas, with seeding of the peritoneum. The surgeon informed the husband that she had less than six months to live. Following the surgery, and unaware of the prognosis, she returned to treatment, where she continued for the next three years. Symptoms were minimal and she chose to stop. Four years later she died from metastases.

2. Lena was a 13-year-old girl with severe ulcerative colitis whose entry into psychoanalytic treatment was precipitated by

the surgeon who stated that after 12 pints of blood, Lena's hemoglobin was only 6 grams and that they were reluctant to do the proposed colectomy. An initial six times a week therapy led to a long-term five times a week analysis, and ultimately into a working alliance and through the conflicts around aggression, dependency, sexuality, and intense issues over control. A long uncooperative period with a stormy transference was present for many, many months. Ultimately, the bleeding stopped, along with the associated symptoms of colitis.

Concomitant with the subsiding of the colitis, was the development of a whole series of overlapping and sequential psychosomatic diseases of decreasing threats to life: asthma, migraine, angioneurotic edema, monoarticular arthritis of the knee, eczema, and nasorhinitis. These symptoms were present alternating with other forms of self-destructive disturbance; depression, automobile accident, and alienation of friends, relatives, and teachers. This self-destructive trajectory of shifting psychosomatic symptoms and self-destructive behavior illustrated that the core problem in this patient's illness was the underlying ego conflict, where insight into the meaning of one syndrome, interferes with its subsequent expression. The partially resolved conflict still required symptomatic representation. After seven years, the ulcerative colitis, and the series of other syndromes, all subsided. A ten-year follow-up consultation revealed no symptoms of ulcerative colitis, or any of those other illnesses. However, she was troubled with pernicious vomiting.

3. Steve was a 29-year-old married engineer, with a history of ulcerative colitis beginning four months after the death of his mother. Salient features in the course of his twice-a-week psychotherapy, reflected his repressed aggression, marked dependency problems, an ambivalent relationship to a controlling mother, conflict in psychosexual identity, and fear of responsibility, the latter epitomized by a terrible fight over having a child.

One evening he had a violent confrontation with his wife over her wish to have a child. That night he developed eight episodes of bleeding, with an accompanying fear that he was bleeding to death. Following an emergency appointment the next morning, further discussion of the conflict resulted in marked physical improvement in the session, with a complete secession of the bleeding when he left. The issues revolved

around his unrecognized anger toward his wife, marked dependency conflict, and issues about his sense of sexual identity and
the wish to have a child. These conflicts resulted in exacerbations
of the colitis and subsequent episodes of bleeding, frequently
on anniversaries.

While the patient developed increasing insight into the nature of his conflicts, with a decrease of symptoms, and increased
assertiveness, and well-being, he was unable to fully resolve his
problems after three-and-one-half years and stopped treatment.

4. Stacey was a 30-year-old librarian in three-times-a-week
analytic psychotherapy. She had a ten-year history of ulcerative
colitis. Symptoms included gas cramps, constipation, and bleeding. She said that she bled so frequently that there was no pro-
tracted period when she did not bleed. She also developed a
monoarticular arthritis of the knee. Her first attack of colitis
occurred six months after the death of her father. On the first-
and second-year anniversaries of his death, the patient developed attacks of colitis so severe that on both occasions she required hospitalization.

Significant conflicts in her life related to an extreme closeness
and ambivalence toward her family, with equivalent levels of
guilt if she did not satisfy what she felt were their needs.

These guilt-filled relationships were masochistic, satisfying
the need to separate and develop her own sense of identity, at
the same time punishing herself for it, and creating problems
in the relationship that precluded their successful conclusion.
Exacerbations of these conflicts resulted in attacks of colitis, and
frequent bleeding. In the fourth month she acted out self-de-
structively with the collusion of her sister and terminated the
treatment.

5. Tom was a 37-year-old married nephrologist, in three-
times-a-week analytic psychotherapy, for a ten-year history of
abdominal pain, diagnosed nine months before treatment as
Crohn's disease. Salient features in his history were a mother,
uncle, and a grandfather all diagnosed with Crohn's disease.

The patient has a close, tumultuous relationship with his
mother, father, younger sister and brother, and his wife, with
early recognition that pressures and conflicts with them resulted
in attacks of abdominal pains and cramps. Strong feelings of
attachment to his family, unassertiveness, and a great deal of

repressed hostility were the major psychodynamic issues he faced. Many episodes of feeling exploited and taken advantage of in social, professional, and family situations all contributed to exacerbations of the pain and cramping.

Although he began to behave more assertively, and recognized the positive effect upon his symptoms, after a year he chose to terminate stating that he felt better, although he was still getting symptoms, and conflicts were still not effectively resolved.

I have seen nine cases in intensive psychoanalytic psychotherapy on a four- to five-session-per-week basis.

One of these patients with Crohn's disease of the colon is still in treatment. He left treatment against medical advice for two years. He returned to treatment two years ago, and remains essentially asymptomatic.

Three other patients with chronic remitting ulcerative colitis have completed psychoanalytic psychotherapy and remain asymptomatic for ten years or more.

One very severe case of Crohn's ileocolitis with multiple perineal, perianal, and abdominal fistulas terminated unimproved after six months. I heard from outside sources that he committed suicide about eighteen months later.

One female patient was much improved and her ulcerative colitis was in remission after two years. But then she developed a severe paranoid transference which we were unable to resolve. She terminated precipitously and I have no follow-up.

One female patient with chronic ulcerative colitis, although much improved, terminated against advice after two years with occasional mild recurrences. Follow-up has indicated very occasional mild colitis attacks when feeling deprived or rejected. These attacks are usually without blood.

One young male patient with Crohn's ileocolitis became asymptomatic and terminated against advice in less than a year of treatment. He did anticipate contacting me if he had further trouble, but I have no follow-up after four years.

For one male patient with chronic ulcerative colitis who would not cooperate in time or attendance and was discharged after two years without remission, I have no follow-up.

In addition to the nine patients above who were in intensive psychoanalytic psychotherapy I have seen three patients, two men and a woman, in less intensive, abbreviated psychotherapy. One remains asymptomatic after more than ten years. The other two are much improved, but do have very occasional mild recurrences and return for short-term treatment.

When we review the results of the treatment of these patients with inflammatory disease of the colon who have been in psychoanalytic psychotherapy we can certainly draw some conclusions. Obviously we are not always completely successful. However, when our results are compared with any series of cases treated with supportive pharmaceutical modalities of therapy, there would seem to be no comparison. We do not consider inflammatory disease of the colon necessarily a life long ailment.

Many psychiatrists and gastroenterologists have recommended supportive psychotherapy over the years. Here I want to call the reader's attention to a difference between "supportive" treatment and intensive short-term analytically oriented psychotherapy.

In psychiatric literature, short-term treatment is often another name of supportive treatment. Each tends to be authoritative but reassuring. On the other hand, short-term psychoanalytic psychotherapy attempts to allow patients the recognition that their problems arise from their own conflicts. Transferential material is used (see chapter 15) to foster an understanding of the dynamics of past conflicts.

As we review the literature of short-term treatment (supportive and otherwise) the results seem to be mixed. I shall present only two studies, but the psychiatric literature is loaded with individual cases. Generally recommendations by gastroenterologists indicate the ancillary nature of supportive supplements.

Weinstock (1966) was most unenthusiastic about results in a series of hospitalized patients. In contrast, Karush et al. (1977) seemed to find rather good results in selected patients in their series.

I believe that most of the members of our Psychosomatic Study Group would join me in agreeing with M. Sperling's position (1969, 1978b). She was opposed to supportive psychotherapy because it immediately brought the unanalyzed primary object (internalized representations of the maternal figure) into the transference. The ambivalence associated with this representation often resulted in a worsening of symptoms.

Many of us wonder if indiscriminate use of supportive treatment is responsible for the occasional cautionary advice of some gastroenterologists about the dangers of psychotherapy with these patients.

As we examine this all too brief review of the literature on the psychoanalytic treatment of inflammatory disease of the colon, there is one feature that presents itself with glaring prominence. There are an astonishing number of incidents of "transference psychosis." A number of investigators have noted this finding occurring most frequently in patients who work it through and go on to recovery. Suffice it to note that at this point we are dealing with patients who repress and suppress very primitive aggression, and who utilize archaic defense mechanisms to deal with such impulses.

Chapter 13
Dynamics and Content

FAMILY BACKGROUND

Consideration of family background is not directly a part of the dynamic study of the patient, it is more in the nature of specialized environmental research; one might include it in an ongoing view of family dynamics. Family history of colitis sufferers yields a fine appreciation of the interrelationships of figures whose mental representations play such a determining role in the fantasied and actual lives of our patients. In our many discussions at The Psychoanalytic Study Group of New York (see Acknowledgments) as well as in my own investigations we have discerned a uniformity in the constellations of individuals with inflammatory disease of the gut. In a larger and less specific sense we have noted a certain uniformity in the families of all psychosomatic patients.

Wilson (1989c) recorded that in our psychosomatic study group

We have investigated the psychological profile in over four hundred psychosomatic families. In a number of psychosomatic families we have detailed (1) the psychoanalytic treatment of psychosomatic patients and the concurrent psychoanalyses of the mother, father, and siblings; (2) the psychodynamic counseling of parents together or separately; (3) the psychoanalytic treatment of a parent, usually the mother; (4) the psychodynamic treatment of the mother and young child; (5) the analyses or analytic psychotherapy of the significant other and the siblings; (6) the unplanned, fortuitous development and/or clearing of psychosomatic symptoms in a significant other or a child in the course of the analysis of a psychosomatic patient or of a non psychosomatic neurotic patient; (7) the supervision of professionals in the treatment of psychosomatic patients [pp. 63–64].

Wilson underlines (pp. 65–67) the family psychopathology of the psychosomatic patient: perfectionism, repression of emotions, infantilizing of decision making, organ-system choice by the family, exhibitionistic parental sexual and toilet behavior and unconscious selection of a particular child for illness are common characteristics of the psychosomatic family.

When treatment begins I see the families of younger patients in consultation. An analyst can often make a fair appraisal of a parent through observation of a patient's subjective representation of the individual family member. There are undoubtedly variations, but I can present reasonably accurate sketches of the typical personalities of mother and father. I can also indicate some of the ways in which these parents uniformly relate to the patient.

The mothers of my colitis patients seem to be somewhat disturbed. Controlling and perfectionistic women who see their children as extensions of themselves, they fear losing control of the child as much as they fear losing control of their own impulses. Their unconscious hostility toward the child is the equivalent of their unconscious destructive self-punitive fantasies about themselves. They may chose one child to play the role of the helpless invalid in their intrapsychic life and that child becomes the colitis sufferer, in my experience, usually the oldest child.

Two of the mothers had difficulty with recurrent diarrhea and bowel preoccupations. One suffered from recurrent constipation. The mother of the Crohn's ileocolitis patient had ulcerative colitis for over thirty years. The mothers' attitudes toward the children's toilet habits, remarkable in every case in that they took positions at either end of the spectrum: some were overcontrolling, others seemed to pay no attention whatsoever to toilet habits. Nevertheless, in all of these families a great deal of verbal attention was directed toward the affairs of the bowel.

Toilet habits and evacuation difficulties of the fathers were more difficult to document without invasive interrogation. However, the father of a patient with Crohn's colitis suffered intermittently from constipation and diarrhea and spent inordinate amounts of time in the bathroom. He constantly medicated himself for hemorrhoids and other anal discomforts. The patient had heard talk of blood so it was difficult to know if his father had an inflammatory process or only hemorrhoids. The father of another patient repeatedly argued with his son as to whether the toilet paper should roll from the top or the bottom.

The fathers of these patients were often professionally accomplished men. Four of them were physicians; the professions of others included writing, journalism, music, and painting. The fathers maintained a rigid morality and vaguely tried to exact the same from their children and spouses. Despite this, a number of interesting contradictions appeared, notable hiatuses in the father's superego development and sense of right and wrong. The father's transgressions were known to the patient, but ostensibly not recognized or acknowledged by the mother; the delinquencies commonly constituted sexual practices: voyeurism, pornography, and varieties of mildly perverse erotic activity with prostitutes. These indulgences of the fathers were reflected in the patients' own perverse fantasies or activities.

The passivity in the father's mildly perverse behavioral deviations extended to the rest of their lives. Despite their accomplishments, they seemed to feel that they had fallen a little short—had failed to accomplish even reasonable ambitions which seemed within their grasp. They repeatedly yielded to their wives and withdrew from any family confrontations. Those who asserted themselves did so with occasional temper tantrums, often when drunk. They all seemed withdrawn from and submissive to their spouses.

The fathers were indulgent of their children, at times distantly so. They were certainly not disciplinarians. Although there was apparent mutual tolerance, there seemed to be a lack of closeness. If I were asked for a character diagnosis, I might judge these fathers as obsessional.

All my male patients began treatment with suppressed but arrogant contempt for their fathers. As treatment progressed repressed affection became more and more evident. The earlier contempt was a reflection of the patient's identification with the suppressed or repressed envy and contempt of the mothers for their husbands.

All in all, the families gave every appearance of closeness. Despite the best of polite familial and social behavior, however, there was a notable lack of mutual affective responses. Jackson and Yalom (1966), in their study of the families of eight patients with ulcerative colitis, noted, "All the families appeared to be severely socially restricted and actively restricted each other in the range of permissible behavior . . . a feeling of despair and yet a feeling of family sameness that almost seemed like solidarity" (p. 418).

Pregenital Conversion

Inflammatory disease of the large bowel has been frequently labeled a pregenital conversion reaction (Deutsch, 1922; Fenichel, 1945a,b). I agree with that designation after allowing for the reservations below and the observations in chapter 9. As noted therein the concept of conversion (Breuer and Freud, 1893–1895, p. 86) has clinically been one of Freud's greatest contributions. The extension of the concept to pregenital conversion has been invaluable to generations of psychoanalytic psychosomaticists (Deutsch, 1922; Fenichel, 1945b; Deutsch and Semrad, 1959; Mushatt, 1954, 1959; M. Sperling, 1963; O. Sperling, 1978a; McDougall, 1982a; Wilson, 1983a; Hogan, 1983a; Mintz, 1989; Sarnoff, 1989).

Over the years investigators have introduced some questions and objections to the concept of pregenital conversion. The first doubt about conversion in general was proposed by Freud himself when he wondered about that "mysterious leap"—the translation of fantasy into physical activity. The second question relates to the fantasies accompanying pregenital conversion reactions. Some observers have questioned the very existence of such fantasies, and if they do exist, their etiological significance. So many aspects of these two questions have been particularized to arguments over the timing of fantasy. It seems difficult to acknowledge dynamic progression or change in content with development. Bertram Lewin was an astute clinician well aware of the dynamic vicissitudes of the fantasy life in the developing individual: "The unconscious meaning of an event depends on its past history and the infantile prototype is usually altered by the processes of development" (1950, p. 135). He recognized that a core affective conflict (with accompanying fantasies) may remain even when its manifest elaborations change as life brings new gratifications and conflicts; and that fantasies appropriate to the original core conflict and to its contemporary elaborations can be in a constant process of change. The recollection of any past fantasy may not be accurate, but in all probability has been contaminated by life's casualties and triumphs, and has amalgamated itself with contemporary perceptions. Psychoanalytic experience has taught us that both recollected and contemporary fantasies reflect the impulses and feelings of past and present.

A patient cannot recall and verbalize a fantasy from a preverbal era. Nonetheless, symptoms, actions, dreams, and associations allow us therapeutically effective reconstructions. In chapter 9 I described a patient who developed an acute "conversion" symptom of masseter spasm followed by a dream of planetary destruction in the context of rage over deprivation. His reconstruction of preverbal rage at the maternal representation was not only therapeutic, it brought repressed reminiscences from a later period of life into consciousness.

It is not too difficult to recognize conflict about, and denial of, conscious sadistic fantasies in the transference and in the social life of a patient. We assume that such impulses and fantasies are ubiquitous in the life of every infant and young child, an assumption based on the content of analyses of adults and children. In the more traditional classic neurotic patient, conflicts over sadism are better integrated, contained, and repressed than in a patient more dependent on pregenital defensive positions. In the psychoneurotic the impulse and fantasy are often integrated into a wish rather than remaining a denied and repressed impulse demanding action. With traditional neurosis conflict between impulse and superego prohibition will appear in a less threatening form later in treatment. In infancy the content of the fantasy is appropriate to that age's experience; if reexperienced in adult life, the content of the fantasy is appropriate to current age and experience. The contemporaneity of fantasy is generally true whether the fantasy is threatening and denied or well integrated into the ego and produced as a psychoanalytic association.

One can observe the age-appropriate quality of content, no matter if the fantasies are sadistically violent, perversely erotic, or mildly benign. The only exceptions seem to be reminiscences of past fantasies and fantasies whose purpose or content require a childish presentation. This quality of appropriateness does not apply to dreams.

As examples, I first present typical fantasies of colitis patients and then focus on those fantasies that parallel the simultaneous cerebral activity that leads to symptoms—historically, the typical pregenital conversion. My review of fantasies does not include the equally typical, but sometimes less frightening, fantasies involving the intense attachment to the primary object. We might also note here that impulses and fantasies of an amorous or erotic nature are shameful and potentially threatening to the colitis patient early in treatment. Such ostensible loss of control is denied, suppressed, and repressed. One male patient eventually admitted that he stayed away from women because involvement brought painful disappointments if he did not feel in complete control of the woman's responses.

The same patient finally volunteered a suppressed chain of associations as to how he constantly amused himself as he rode the subway or walked down the street. He would pick some male of a different ethnic background and then fantasy that the man approached and insulted or challenged him as he aggressively and sarcastically responded to the challenge. The fantasied violence and rhetoric escalated, turning into a physical confrontation: he would pull out his knife and his adversary would either have a knife or a gun. The patient oscillated between two endings: in one he emerged victorious standing above a humiliated and mutilated, or dead, victim; in the other my patient was the humiliated and mutilated, or dead, victim. After obsessive rumination, he usually preferred the latter version, and proceeded to another, similar fantasy. Equally ferocious scenarios were manufactured with the mildest of social confrontations. As a matter of fact, they accompanied the majority of his social interchanges. The fantasies were present-day reenactments of fantasies and actions directed against (and, of course, intense homoerotic involvement with) his younger brothers and father during his oedipal and early latency years. The availability of the primitive violence was derivative of pregenital conflicts. The content seemed to reflect the quality of his self-destructive accident-proneness that began at a remarkably early age—late infancy. The polymorphous perverse nature of primitive attachments was reflected in his preoccupation with similar mental dialogues with women who interested him. One would humiliate the other, sometimes with elaborate sexual activity. These subjective scenarios often ended up in violence and rape by him and/or violent cruelty and/or rejection by the woman. I have already referred to his profound fear of involvement and shame at admitting affectionate feelings. The suppressed but still more available sadism was defensively a regressive move from any admission of tender erotic interest. I should note that in the early phases of treatment this patient carried a knife.

A female ulcerative colitis patient was in psychoanalytic psychotherapy for two years before she admitted to repeated "amusing" transference fantasies that had preoccupied her since the first weeks of treatment: she would either knock down my bookcases, shove me out the window, physically attack my genitals, or burn the building. The fantasies replicated infantile (2 to 3 years) fantasies of tearing down or burning her house as well as other fantasies of attacking or burning her mother or sister. As one might guess, these two were ultimately perceived as regressive defenses against erotic transferential interests.

Colitis patients' violent defensive fantasy and dream material are par for the course once the patient has acknowledged and worked through some of the fear of verbalizing associations that are repugnant to the ego. The male colitis patient mentioned above, whenever threatened, could manufacture sadistic dissection fantasies of infinite variety involving either himself or the offending other.

Harold Levitan (1976, 1977, 1978, 1981, 1982, 1989a,b) has contributed a great deal of material from his studies of successive cases of psychosomatic illness with an interest in impulses, dreams, precipitating circumstances, and the ego's defensive functions in psychosomatic patients. His work confirms statistically what we see clinically in the psychoanalytic treatment of colitis patients. He observed the rage and the lack of object relatedness in the etiology and the onset of ulcerative colitis (1976, 1977, 1989a), accumulating interesting material on the prevalence of violent themes and incest motifs in the dreams of psychosomatic patients (1982, 1989b), in whom he indicates a failure in the defensive functions of the ego (1981, 1989b). My own emphasis would be on the regression in the ego with primitive impulses opposed by equally primitive superego precursors, but our differences might be in emphasis and description. Nevertheless, Levitan's extensive observations reveal material that is substantially the same as that revealed in the fantasies and dreams of patients in psychoanalysis or psychoanalytic psychotherapy.

We now address those fantasies simultaneously parallel to the cerebral activity that initiates and maintains the physiological forces responsible for the symptoms of inflammatory colitis.

A young male patient with Crohn's of the descending colon and rectum had been ill for seven years and the current severe exacerbation was of six months' duration. His physician had warned him and his parents that without surgery he would die. Within one week, this for the most part bedridden, cachectic, and emaciated young man was telling of fears of impulses he had had to murder a former friend who he felt had humiliated him. The subjective awareness of colitis and its accompanying immobilization was preferable to what he felt would be insanity and murder. He unconsciously (often consciously) welcomed a pregenital conversion—the severe exacerbation in his Crohn's colitis. The fantasies of colitis patients very often display a primitive quality of urgency. The patient experiences an impulse that demands gratification and is afraid either of acting on the taboo drive or being thought crazy for entertaining the unbidden, unleashed craving.

A young female patient had gone through some traumatic life experiences, including a brother's recent suicide. She had been in a constant state of rage at and envy of the attention given to him before his suicide, and had an unusually intense conscious resentment of her younger sister. She had left the family to support herself shortly before the brother's death, and developed her colitis some months after. She was aware of her own fantasies and the conflict over her impulses and fears at the time she began psychoanalytic psychotherapy, but in the familiar manner of colitis patients she was able to split off, deny, and suppress the material without acknowledging that she was holding back associations. Eventually we recovered her fantasies about her brother's suicide. She had often fantasied his destruction or castration, but that seemed less important than her conclusion that since her brother was dead she would get more attention and might even be asked to return to the family home. Instead she felt forced to sympathize with her grief-stricken, withdrawn, and self-centered parents who seemed to show no interest in her or her problems. In her suppressed rageful fantasies she considered family destruction on the one hand and her own suicide on the other. She compromised with the partial suicide of subjectively experiencing ulcerative colitis and its accompanying preconscious fantasies of the sadistic destruction of her family, and of course of herself. This material appeared at a much later date when she began to forfeit the experience of her symptoms. As she gave up her symptoms, her fantasy and dream life repeatedly involved shitting out or on various representations of family members, material not initially suggested or interpreted. With great concern over her own sanity she finally volunteered these dreams along with others of a cannibalistic nature. Associations led back to fantasies about the brother's birth and her infantile oral ideas of impregnation and conception.

Her dream content paralleled her fantasy life. In one dream she looked in the toilet bowl and saw dolls instead of feces. Her associations went to her sister. In another, there was a bloody scene of a cat having kittens, leading back to observations in childhood of her cat giving birth, which in turn brought up existent fantasies (remembrances?) of her sister's birth.

We know from generations of psychoanalytic experience that the manifest content of dream or fantasy is of less importance than the associations. We also know that repeated representation of primitive impulse and conflict in the manifest content of dreams and fantasies is usually indicative of regressive disturbances. The drives and defenses are remnants of pregenital times but are often amalgamated with phallic or oedipal concerns. Erotism, sadism, and masochism are fused. When a patient relinquishes a severe psychosomatic symptom such as inflammatory colitis, one commonly observes its replacement with another psychosomatic symptom or a succession of them. One unusual example was Mintz's patient (see p. 145) who during treatment displayed sequentially: ulcerative colitis, asthma, migraine, angioneurotic edema, monoarticular arthritis of the knee, eczema, and nasorhinitis. A second remarkable example was described by Levitan (1978), whose patient manifested in succession: bronchial asthma, peptic ulcer, regional ileitis, and anorexia nervosa. Inflammatory colitis patients not uncommonly progress to, or temporarily interrupt, the colitis with symptomatic expressions like eczema, tension headaches, or migraine headaches. One patient of mine developed a mild transient self-limited right-sided hemiparesis with slurring of speech and all the characteristic neurological signs.

In chapter 2 I listed a number of associated pathological conditions and complications that can accompany ulcerative colitis and Crohn's disease of the colon. Some may be in the nature of conversion reactions and many may be secondary to the physically disabling effects of recurrent exacerbations of gut disease. I want to direct attention to two associated conditions that were not listed in that chapter since they too seem to qualify as accompanying pregenital conversions. They may be a part of the same process. The first might be approached as an isolated conversion reaction or as an extension of the conversion reactions in the gastrointestinal tract. The second seems clearly to represent a separate pregenital conversion.

The first associated symptom is the appearance of a bluish pallor to the lips (cyanosis?), upon which three of my patients commented, volunteering that this often precedes an attack of colitis, but can occasionally occur without an attack. The sign seems to be almost always related to the internal psychic conflict likely to be associated with the initiation of an attack (two ulcerative colitis, one Crohn's colitis). The second associated condition appeared in four of my patients, characterized by attacks of hyperhidrosis and/or bromhidrosis, bouts of excessive and often malodorous perspiration which did not usually accompany attacks of colitis but seemed to replace them. In two cases the attacks were particularly noticeable when the patients were giving up their colitis symptoms. They evinced the same intense overt shame and embarrassment accompanying the colitis, yet their associations, fantasies, and dreams led to the same rebellious pleasures of impulsively offending and contaminating the environment so characteristic in the sadistic world of the colitis patient. These episodes of acrid perspiration seemed to disappear, or at least become infrequent, as the patients went into remission.

OBJECT RELATIONS

The major initiating problems in the psychoanalytic psychotherapy of colitis patients are in the realms of their defensive pregenital postures, and here we are intimately involved with those ubiquitous internalizations of fragmented object representations.

Charles Brenner (1979a) noted: "I may say in passing that what is valid in so-called object relations theory seems to me to involve substituting a new term—object relations—for a familiar one—drive derivative" (p. 554), and I have no disagreement with his defense of the drive–conflict theory. However, I am not sure that we are dealing with conflicting theories. If we ignore other Kleinian formulations, are we not dealing generally with levels or orders of abstraction? The advantage of discussing drive derivatives in terms of object relations is that we are dealing with a lower order of abstraction—one that can often be translated into terms that the patient can eventually understand. It is easy enough to interpret object representations as feelable "ghosts of the past" represented in contemporary perceptions of projections. The patient can present his mental scenarios of contemporary objects, and with reasonable ease see them as representations of past objects or part objects. On the other hand, the concept of drive derivative is a more generalized descriptive phrase for a much higher order of abstraction in psychoanalytic observation and theory. It is a useful theoretical construct but not as demonstrable or useful in physician–patient communication.

The ego of the colitis patient is not only poorly differentiated from the perceptions of the contemporary and the primitive object, but is also poorly differentiated within itself. Figuratively, it is riddled by fragmented judgmental part objects, traditionally precursors of the more mature and differentiated superego. These patients live in a world of judgment, of right and wrong. In turn they are judgmental of their object perceptions, which contain all of their own projective identifications. They do not usually verbalize such judgments for fear of their own judgmental superegos, which anticipate humiliation, punishment, and abandonment.

The lack of acknowledgment of separation from contemporary objects is reflected in the projective identification and the feeling in many of these patients that they know what the object is thinking. This in turn leads to the patient's need for the illusion of control over self and object.

Object Relations: The Need for Control

M. Sperling (1961, 1967, 1968) has emphasized the psychosomatic patient's need for control as often as has any observer. It is interesting that she saw her patients' use of their objects as fetishes to control rather than as people to have feelings about. Colitis patients sustain a subjective certainty that they must, and are expected to be, in control of their own feelings, thoughts, and associations at all times. In the transference this is reflected in the intense shame associated with any evidence of loss of control, whether the loss involves anal or erotic material, verbal expressions of aggression, recognition of needs or wants, or associated fears of abandonment. Concomitant with the compulsion to control their own feelings is the automatic need to control (their perceptions of) the object (projection). (The details of the specific need to control the treatment and the psychoanalyst are discussed in chapters 15 and 16 on transference and countertransference.) It is not difficult to understand "alexithymia" in the early treatment of many of these patients. They cannot avoid feeling that psychoanalysis or psychoanalytic therapy is an authoritative study of the rules of the game and that their job is to learn what is right or wrong and how to behave appropriately.

The need for control is often one aspect of an obsessional character structure with a lack of spontaneity. There are marked fears and inhibitions of all impulse indulgences—except for colonic needs, in which case the patients feel totally out of control. We should note at this point that none of these patients has much freedom of sexual expression. The women are unable to have orgasm with intercourse. Many are orgastic with manual or oral manipulation, but some unconsciously insist on maintaining unconscious control even over these potentially orgastic expressions. Males are commonly able to perform sexually, but usually get very little sexual pleasure from their performance. They have premature ejaculations, betraying one area where control is lost, and tremendous unconscious fear of a relationship with the sexual object.

Fortunately, the patient's rigidity is usually not so severe as to permanently mediate against treatment. As the psychoanalytic therapy progresses these individuals are capable of a greater spontaneity. As a matter of fact, as the symptoms are given up, there are intermittent periods of indulgence. Acting out is an almost universal phase of successful treatment.

OBJECT RELATIONS: FRAGMENTATION

An inadequate sense of separation from the object is reflected in projective mechanisms and invariably accompanied by splitting (see chapters 15 and 16). From the object relations point of view, splits are accompaniments of unconscious identifications—infantile internalizations of part object representations—multiple identifications carrying the threat of conscious fragmentation and playing an important role in the need for an illusory sense of control.

Freud (1923) acknowledged this state of affairs when he spoke of "the ego's object identifications. If they obtain the upper hand and become too numerous, unduly powerful and incompatible with one another, a pathological outcome will not be far off" (p. 30). "At the very beginning, in the individual's primitive oral phase, object-cathexis and identification are no doubt indistinguishable from each other . . . the character of the ego is a precipitate of abandoned object-cathexes and it contains the history of those object-choices" (p. 29). He continued: "it may come to a disruption of the ego in consequence of the different identifications becoming cut off from one another by resistances . . . . [E]ven when things do not go so far as this, there remains the question of conflicts between the various identifications into which the ego comes apart" (p. 30–31). Heimann (1942) discussed a patient whose multiple "devils" evidently represented separate internalized part objects in a fantasied form. (See Niederland's [1956, 1965] "little man" and Volkan's [1965, 1975] "stick man" for examples of representations of such isolated fragmented part objects.)

Unlike pregenital fragmentation (Hogan, 1983b, pp. 143–144) in patients with anorexia nervosa, patients with inflammatory disease of the colon do not, before treatment, demonstrate conscious confusion and are not usually subjectively conscious of splitting. Paradoxically, the less regressed anorexic patients seem to have a greater ability to tolerate uncontrolled fragmentation and consequently occasionally tolerate the symptomatic expression of the confusion. Some anorexia-bulimia patients take a certain pride in exposing their "flibberty-gibbet" confusion, but most colitis patients would be mortified by any display of loss of control.

In the colitis patient, on the other hand, the fragmentation becomes apparent as treatment progresses and the patient reveals his separate identifications. For the most part, the repressed fragmentation remains a potential threat and is extremely frightening when it does break through. A barely suppressed awareness of instability seems to play a part in the colitis patient's frequent fear of being crazy. One patient of mine, as treatment progressed, was well aware of his multiple identifications. He protected himself from subjective chaos by obsessively scrutinizing his separate ego states. He spoke of conflicting "levels" of thought and conflicting "outlooks," progressing through scenarios of contradictions. The obsessional developing awareness of isolated identifications is not uncommon in colitis patients.

One can recognize similarities in the pregenital defenses, with their fragmented object relations, in all psychosomatic patients. The defenses take on somewhat different manifestations depending on the specific level of psychosomatic regression. In occasional very regressed patients, transference psychoses appear (see chapter 12).

OBJECT RELATIONS: OMNIPOTENCE

A primitive sense of omnipotence accompanying all of these part self/part object representations is experienced either as an identification and part of the self or as a projection and a quality of the contemporary object.

As a quality of the self the sense of omnipotence plays a part in the need for immediate gratification and/or immediate action. Colitis patients are terrified of their impulses and react to their perceived potential dangers as though the impulses and wishes might magically and omnipotently be gratified. There is also a quality of omnipotence and omniscience in the colitis patient's certainty that he or she knows what the important object is thinking and how it is judging. A sense of omnipotence is always present in projection or projective identification. In early symptomatic periods with regressive defenses, the patient has little if any conscious awareness of this sense of omnipotence, he experiences projections and identifications as natural parts of an undifferentiated self and feels that omnipotent incorporation of objects is what the world is all about. Until immersion in psychoanalytic psychotherapy the patient is unaware of his or her "separateness."

An increasing awareness of an elated omnipotence develops as the patient gives up subjective representations of the physical symptoms (along with the symptom) and begins to act out. Now the patient slowly notices the elated omnipotent fantasy of overcoming the superego (Lewin, 1950) when indulging in some action that is perceived as forbidden, an action containing the potential for self-punishment. Any awareness of potential danger is unconscious while the elation is conscious, but may be temporarily denied.

One of my patients, during a period of acting out and in the process of understanding this defense, presented an interesting dream:

> I was on the top of the Pan Am building [helicopter landing area at that time] and began to run excitedly in circles. I was thrilled and elated—finally I just sailed off the edge of the building, fell down through space in a panic and I guess I crashed into the ground.

The situational associations are not important for our purposes, but in the manifest content of this dream we can see the patient's awakening to his conflict about his wish for elated action and his fear of the punishing consequences involved, either in fantasy or reality. The sexual implications of the dream are also clear, but these are in the context of an entirely different level of development; they are not a preconscious part of the patient's contemporary conflicts and associations. This material has to be interpreted and discussed in terms of the immediate regressed preoccupations of omnipotence, elation, action, and control; and not in the context of the still quite repressed sexual spheres of unconscious conflict.

One can easily see how the omnipotence is projected upon the perceived object as one follows the transference. These patients are certain of omnipotent and omniscient moral judgments by the analyst. Thoughts of the analyst reading the patient's mind are not uncommon. Similarly, intermittently denied ideas that the analyst perceives the patient's motivation without the patient's informative associations are almost universal.

In my discussion of the sense of omnipotence, I am not referring to the completely regressed omnipotent omniscient oceanic fantasy of oneness with the universe that is often cited as a manifestation of psychoses and some religious experiences. I am speaking of the related defensive use of omnipotence first clearly discussed by Riviere (1936) in her paper "A Contribution to the Analysis of a Negative Therapeutic Reaction." She described the omnipotent elated organized system of defense that in Kleinian terms she labeled "manic" and saw as used against the "depressive position." She also emphasized that it was a defense aimed at warding off depression and guilt over primitive sadistic impulses.

Lewin (1950) contributed much to understanding the affects associated with the fantasied reunion with mother (i.e., reunion of ego and id with the superego). It is a tribute to Lewin, and a since neglected area of the pleasure principle, that he contributed so much and that so little has been written about the elation involved in all regressive disturbances (and reunions). It is also too bad that more has not been written on elation as the affective component of omnipotence.

My observations of the omnipotent fantasies experienced and the elations felt in the regressive defenses and activities of colitis patients are not new. The major difficulty has been others' evident lack of interest in working with patients who display psychosomatic symptoms and in understanding the vicissitudes of early infantile fantasies and affects, an avoidance particularly striking when treating inflammatory gut disease.

SYMPTOM FORMATION

Any study of parallel subjective dynamics, including parallel cerebral changes contributing to the reversibility of colonic disease, in no way contradicts the extensive research of the mechanics, chemistry, and anatomical pathophysiology of the colon and colonic disease processes. The study of the control of the hypothalamo-pituitary-adrenocortical axis is not in opposition to, nor a contradiction of, the psychoanalytic study of patients with inflammatory disease of the colon.

I approach the subject of symptom formation as a follow-up of my discussions of pregenital conversions and object relations. The physical symptoms of ulcerative colitis and Crohn's disease parallel pregenital defensive problems involving relationships with perceived projections and projective identifications of primitive part object representations. The major physical symptoms are traditionally identified as pregenital conversion phenomena.

I have already discussed the regression and/or fixation of these patients to or at a primitive level of development, in which there is a repressed need for immediate gratification, and an impulse to immediate action if gratification is denied. There are complementary defenses against these needs and impulses and their projected representations. The affects accompanying frustration of needs and impulses include exquisite humiliation and retaliatory sadistic impulses to control and destroy; the affects and impulses are invariably accompanied by content—fantasy. The original fantasies as well as the contemporary ones are usually repressed, but one finds that contemporary fantasies (transference fantasies are good examples) about current perceptions of projected object representations are often suppressed or barely concealed in the preconscious.

Recognizing that any number of explanatory interpretations may be imposed on any observable clinical finding, I have contributed one minor complication in my demonstration that the data of subjective productions of symptoms are not in themselves causative—it merely parallels other data, cerebral activity, neurological and physiological processes that are part of a causal chain. However, I have also demonstrated that the acceptance of one set of data in no way compromises or interferes with the acceptance of data from the other observational platform. When we speak of mind or brain we are speaking of different sets of data that often represent an identity.

We observe clinically the patient's contributions that equate their physical symptoms with their own sadistic fantasies of devouring and excreting fantasied enemies and ultimately representations of the primary object. There are all of the recognized anal sadistic fantasies about contemporary and historical

objects—"shitting on" and all of its variations and synonyms—and all of the forcible sexual variations of "up yours."
The prevalence of sadistic anal language and fantasy is shared
with other patients with pregenital and anal problems. The
fantasies and dreams unique to colitis patients seem to include
oral cannibalistic material with intestinal churning and anal
elimination of cannibalistically incorporated objects.

Now, were such specific fantasies present in the pregenital
and even preverbal area of development characteristic of this
level of regression? I should think not. The fantasies these
patients verbalize are too evolved and sophisticated in their
content to be direct memories or representations of the content
of that undifferentiated level of development. We do have reason to believe, however, that the fantasies are contemporary
representations of whatever subjective states accompanied
these angry sadistic affective states of the oral and anal period
of development. The fantasies are also contemporary representations of those earlier fears of losing the ambivalently experienced object. As clinicians, our observations confirm that our
patients' recognition, verbalization, and resolution of conflicts
about sadistic impulses and their accompanying fantasies allow
for a resolution of the symptoms of bloody colitis in the parallel
physiological area of data retrieval. When we clinicians can see
a repeated demonstration of a relationship, we have no choice
but to report our data and draw the obvious conclusions.

In the subjective (fantasy) world of the patient, the mental
representations of colonic activity represent the fantasy of an
action taken on an object, which may be a contemporary derivative of the representation of an infantile object. When conflict
about sadistic impulses (and accompanying fantasies) toward
an ambivalently experienced loved object is acknowledged and
resolved, the patient is able to give up the subjective representation of colonic activity (along with the pathophysiology of colitis). Usually at this juncture the need to gratify impulses is not
resolved to the point of analyzing the infantile nature of the
impulse. Consequently, a period of acting out usually follows

(and overlaps) symptomatic activity. The acting out also seems to represent the same omnipotent sadistic fantasies of control that were such an important part of the impulse gratification reflected in the symptoms.

Any psychoanalytic observer will recognize the oversimplicity of the abstractions presented here. What about the overdetermination of the symptoms and the action? A compromise formation in both symptom and acting out assures the superego that the participant is adequately punished for his hidden impulses, whether the punishment lies in the symptoms or in the results of the acting out. When patients work out their pregenital conflicts they progress to a higher level of development, in which self-punishment takes the form of subjective guilt and the analyst is at last working with the depressions and/or phobias of a more traditional psychoneurosis. Here again there is an oversimplification in my abstraction. The progression, while traceable, is never so neat, but consists of leaps forward and repeated regressions. These patients have utilized denial in its various forms as a principal defense, and we can observe that colitis patients utilize it in all phases of treatment to a greater extent than do more traditional psychoneurotics.

We have a lot more to learn about symptom formation and the parallel sets of data presented in the parallel languages of the subjective self and the observed physical being. We are certain, however, that in a reasonable percentage of the patient population, we can see a reversal in the symptomatology and prolonged remissions. In an ideal setting where psychoanalytic therapy is available, this form of treatment would appear to have advantages over other therapeutic approaches.

I would hope that in our contemporary medical world, where science seems to be equated with mechanical technological progress, enough truly scientific psychoanalytic practitioners will become interested in the facts of data collection—the accumulation of data (facts) about the patient's subjective self paralleling the data (facts) about the externally viewed physical self—to help us communicate these greater dimensions of medical understanding.

OEDIPAL CONCERNS IN TREATMENT

FIXATION OR REGRESSION

The symptom complex of ulcerative colitis and Crohn's disease of the colon is associated with the vicissitudes of pregenital conflict. Since these findings seem to be a reaffirmation of consistent psychoanalytic observations over the last half century, it is apparent that we are dealing with either a regression from oedipal conflict or a fixation at an early level of development.

In my opinion, it is difficult to evaluate in individual cases the degree of fixation as opposed to the degree of regression. An assumption is usually made that fixation implies a constitutional defect arising from a genetic or developmental arrest. This to some would indicate an unfortunate condition that carries with it either the impossibility of a developmental change or at best the need for difficult manipulation involving some form of psychological replacement therapy.

If we were to assume that the severity of the physical symptoms reflects the degree of fixation as opposed to the degree of regression, we would be at a loss to prove our point. In order to evaluate our assumption we would hypothesize that the greater the degree of fixation the less the possibility of reversing the disease process. In my case series, and in the psychoanalytic literature, the severity of the disease process seems to have little correlation with the probability of prolonged remission or recovery.

I do not feel that there is a clear-cut separation between fixation and regression. I believe that, as with most biological and psychological phenomena, the observer witnesses a complex multidimensional blend of constitutional predispositions, developmental (familial environmental) vicissitudes and conflicts, and precipitating preconditions. Psychosomatic patients often have a predispositional early developmental conflict with the mother or surrogate. This may arise partially in the context of genetic and constitutional predispositions and/or it may be in reaction to the personality conflicts of the maternal figure. Again, as with most biological and psychological continua, it probably represents both. When providing a background for triadic sexual conflict in the phallic and oedipal areas of concern, the early fixation would seem to present a rallying point for defense in regression from oedipal problems. Only such a complexity of developmental conflicts would explain our clinical findings in the subjective world of the colitis patient.

The oedipal conflicts that these patients are defending against (have regressed from) run the gamut of oedipal concerns. When patients with inflammatory bowel disease give up their pregenital defensive postures we see the usual presentation of phallic and oedipal conflicts. There are always some severe depressive concerns and often the development of phobic symptomatology.

It is important to discover the colitis patient's sexual interests and inhibitions at the initiation of treatment and to know a little of his or her sexual development.

SEXUAL DEVELOPMENT

All my female patients were orgastically unresponsive to intercourse at the beginning of treatment. One young woman can be presented as a typical example of the fears, defenses, and inhibitions characteristic of female colitis patients. She revealed a history of compromised childhood impulse control of a mildly perverse nature. As a preschool child she had an erotic interest in defecating in public places, where she was not observed, but where her products would be discovered. There was no known unusual history of nocturnal enureses, but poor daytime bladder control was still present at the initiation of

treatment. When excited she often urinated, and had had ex-
cruciatingly shameful losses of bladder control at times when
one would expect sexual arousal such as petting experiences
with a boyfriend.

Male patients seem to engage in compulsive sexual activity,
but infrequently and badly, without a great deal of sexual pleasure. They often rationalize the shortfall by an ostensibly strict
moral behavioral stance. Others have little or no heterosexual
activity. A patient presented adolescent and adult masturbation
fantasies typical of a male colitis patient with voyeuristic and
exhibitionistic content and behavior. As his analysis progressed,
early memories of manually dilating his anus and showing it
off to other children came to light. One of his favorite pastimes
at the ages of 3 and 4 was to run from home naked, exhibiting
himself and particularly his anus through the neighborhood.
This material was recalled with intense humiliation. Later,
memories of equally intense erotic pleasure were also recovered.

Those patients who remain in treatment and gain a successful resolution of their organic symptoms begin to wrestle with
the typical phallic and oedipal problems of sexual identification
and erotic attachments. Against the depressions and phobias
that then appear in this compulsive group of people, denial
seems to remain a frequently utilized posture of defense. Along
with denial, acting out of sexual conflict is perhaps a greater
problem in this group of patients than it is in the more typical
and traditional psychoneurotic patient. In patients seemingly
devoted to marital partners, eruptions of extramarital interests
and activities are extremely common. Not infrequently an interest in mild forms of heterosexual perversion is awakened. Earlier in treatment, at the time of resolution of organic symptoms,
self-destructive acting out is extremely common, but it is usually
not of an overtly sexual nature. Sexual acting out characteristic
of the later stage of treatment, in my experience, is quite circumscribed in its nature. While it may put a romance or marriage in jeopardy, it does not seem to be an attempt to provoke
physical or social retribution.

INITIATING ENVIRONMENTAL CONDITIONS

Much has been written on bereavement and separation as initiating conditions for colitis and other psychosomatic (as well as "organic") syndromes. The use of the term *bereavement* has a certain pragmatic utility for the observer who has withdrawn from the psychoanalytic subjective observational areas. It has accumulated meanings beyond those of subjective experience. It is applied epidemiologically to any inferred loss of relationship, regardless of what that loss might mean to the concerned individual. Not surprisingly, there is some *statistical* conformity, as one might expect. In all the literature on bereavement virtually no one refers to the variety of meanings of the word in the variety of contexts in which it is used (as with the word *stress*). In all of the discussion and speculation about the statistical findings there is an assumed and unwarranted identity attributed to a term whose definition has grown to take on a number of meanings and contexts other than the original context of subjective feeling.

In the individual subjective worlds of our colitis patients there does seem to be a specific vulnerability to the loss of a perceived constellation matching an internalized representation of the primary object, which may be a human, an environmental constellation, an environmental parameter, an ideal or can, as at times in epidemiological studies, be a parent, other relative, spouse, or surrogate. But we must also note that the loss often represents a loss of control over the object. The devastation incurred depends on the subjective meaning of the lost situation or object. In any case, the loss is more than a depressing loss of a loved object or abstraction. It denotes a loss of a fantasy of control over an ambivalently experienced relationship. A lost parent or spouse is not a devastating loss of control over an object for every individual or even for every colitis patient (although in any series of patients it may be statistically significant). The important scientific issue is the subjective meaning of the specific event to the individual. If one utilizes the term *bereavement* it should be used in its original sense of subjective sense of loss. It has little meaning once it is expanded, with inferred subjective meaning, to include every objectively witnessed departure of a supposedly needed object. Any statistical study that assumes a universal meaning for an assumed environmental provocation begins with a profound error.

Nevertheless, as in all regressed patients, the onset of symptoms is often precipitated by a sense of loss or abandonment with all of its conscious and unconscious ramifications to that particular individual.

COMPARATIVE OUTCOME

With a series of cases as short as mine, or for that matter that of most psychoanalysts, it is hard to reach any generalizations about outcomes of successfully treated colitis patients as compared to successfully treated psychoneurotic patients, but I will try. (See Weinstock's series, chapter 12.)

Treated psychosomatic patients, compared to treated psychoneurotic patients, are inclined to display more energetic, perhaps aggressive, ambition once they have resolved the inhibitions of their anger. Although other psychosomatic patients may display various character traits from the hysterical to the obsessional, all of my colitis patients seemed to retain a rather obsessional attitude toward life and work.

It is gratifying to both patient and analyst to recognize that one can, with reasonable success, reduce or eliminate subjective representations as well as physical symptoms of inflammatory disease of the colon.

Chapter 14
Technical Considerations

INTAKE PROCEDURES

In the treatment of cases with psychosomatic symptoms (Hogan, 1990) one is frequently faced with certain pregenital defenses and conflicts that call upon the intuition and ingenuity of the psychoanalyst to enlist the patient in the psychoanalytic process. "Conventional psychoanalytic wisdom teaches us that treatment and its modifications are dictated by the nature of the underlying neurosis or psychosis regardless of the symptom" (p. 229). We find in some psychosomatic cases a clear, identifiable psychoneurosis, a character disorder, a definable borderline condition, or a psychotic regression. This is not usually the case in patients with inflammatory disease of the colon. We have seen that C. D. Murray (1930b) and A. J. Sullivan (1935), as well as numerous other early investigators, indicated the absence of identifying psychiatric symptoms when the patient first enters treatment. The psychic pain is usually not mentioned in the early interviews, unless the investigator inquires into subjective symptomatology. Even when such an inquiry is initiated, psychological symptoms are frequently denied.

Some patients display denial to such a degree that an entire hierarchy of emotional conflicts ranging from serious pregenital difficulties to doubts about sexual identity and oedipal concerns may be hidden and subsumed in the organic symptom. Any clear evaluation of the psychiatric diagnosis is usually impossible in the beginning phase of therapy. When the denial is relinquished (and/or when the psychosomatic symptom is temporarily given up) we are able to see the patient's rather primitive intense dyadic transference attachment and we can begin to understand the evolving psychopathology and accompanying psychological symptomatology.

When the psychoanalyst first encounters a patient with inflammatory disease of the gut, he must remember that the patient has potentially life-threatening symptoms demanding certain parameters unnecessary in the treatment of the psychoneuroses. The extent of the parameters and the nature of the analyst's direct involvement will depend upon the pathophysiology of the colon. The more acute and life-threatening the symptoms, the greater the need for immediate intervention. It is necessary to combine investigative procedures from a pathophysiological and from a psychoanalytic viewpoint in a clinical setting that will allow for future interpretable psychoanalytic work and an interpretable transference relationship.

In my own experience supervising other psychoanalysts, it is in the early phase of the treatment process that therapy is likely to reach a stalemate or at times a crisis, sometimes requiring physical intervention, and it is exactly at this point in treatment that supportive psychotherapy can be most destructive. If the psychoanalyst becomes reassuring and supportive, he or she is communicating to the patient the therapist's anxiety about the patient's condition. This is likely to mobilize all of the patient's primitive, as yet unanalyzed, ambivalence toward the mother (introjected representation). The patient's somatic compliance with the accompanying masochistic activity is likely to further aggravate an already serious situation. I shall offer clinical material below, but for the moment, let us stay with a discussion of the general principles of handling the initial phases of treatment.

Are we allowed to presume that, when a psychoanalyst avoids any group of patients, we are dealing with a countertransference problem? As Otto Sperling (1978b) indicated, many psychoanalysts are willing to speculate about and develop theories on the genesis and mechanisms of psychosomatic disorders, but few have been willing to engage in their psychoanalytic treatment. Some expand their studies beyond the realm of psychosomatics to the all-inclusive spheres of biopsychosocial studies. Others refuse to acknowledge the existence of any psychopathology in patients in whom we recognize psychosomatic symptoms.

One can actually observe a fear of taking on the responsibility of treating a patient with destructive and life-threatening symptoms like inflammatory pathology of the large bowel. When the interested psychoanalytic physician is careful, as well as emotionally and intellectually prepared, there is every reason that, with adequate training, he or she should feel free to exercise acumen and talent in this field.

Giovacchini (1975, 1979b) discussed the role of the analyst's countertransference in judging the suitability of a patient for psychoanalysis. Boyer (1961, 1979) suggested that unresolved countertransference reactions may constitute the major obstacle to the successful treatment of patients with serious characterological disorders, noting (1979): "that it is difficult to define and delineate one's inner experiences on one's technical and tactical maneuvers [with characterological and schizophrenic disorders]. Few analysts beyond Searles [1963, 1966, 1975, 1979] and to a lesser degree Giovacchini have sought to do so" (pp. 348–349). Boyer uses his own inner experiences to illustrate countertransference reactions to projective identifications (1979, pp. 347–374).

Psychosomatic patients in general, and individuals with inflammatory bowel disease in particular, have a special barrier between themselves and the possibility of treatment by a psychoanalyst. Although most physicians will at least acknowledge that the treatment of characterological problems and schizophrenic disorders lies in the professional area of psychiatry, few hold this view with regard to psychosomatic disorders. Probably the majority of involved internists and surgeons deny that the symptoms of these patients have any relationship to parallel psychological conflicts. In the case of inflammatory disease of the gut, this majority is quite vocal in its disparagement of psychoanalytic, or even psychiatric, interference.

This situation contributes to the reluctance of many psychoanalysts to become involved in the controversy. Incidentally, it
also contributes some difficulty to the task of the psychoanalyst
when he tries to find a cooperative and understanding internist
or surgeon. Such resistance keeps many patients from seeking
or finding psychoanalytic treatment.

In inflammatory bowel disease we are dealing with potentially debilitating and, not infrequently, life-threatening symptoms. While some feel that our approach may contradict the
traditional psychoanalytic passivity, it is important to obtain a
careful medical and psychiatric history of treatment medications, and hospitalizations with whatever relevant documenta-
tion one feels is necessary.

It is also important to establish contact with a consultant
internist and/or surgeon, the timing of which in treatment,
again, depends upon the nature and severity of the initiating
symptomatology.

These patients often have been seen and treated by practitioners who neglect and/or deny the importance of, or are
downright hostile toward, the intervention of a physician interested in the observation of the subjective emotional aspects of
the conflicts paralleling the genesis and continuation of pathophysiological colonic activity. It is important that the patient
tell us about the attitudes of previous clinicians and the patient's
feelings about past experiences, but it is not wise to challenge
directly or argue about past professional recommendations. As
in the more traditional analytic interview, the physician should
remain noncommittal. Only later does one raise tentative questions.

New patients not uncommonly are on one or more medications. Unless there is an obvious medical reason, the psychoanalyst or the consultant should not immediately interfere. At some
time in the early stages of treatment it is ordinarily advisable
to communicate to patients that it is our mutual expectation
that they will eventually discover that the gut is under their
own control, and that their medications are treating only the

symptoms. One can as time goes by and, with medical consultation if necessary, find that patients suggest decreasing medication. There is one clear danger at this moment: no patient
should precipitously stop medication with steroids.

PRIMARY PHYSICIAN

This brings us to a frequent and most important point of
controversy with our medical and surgical colleagues on the
one hand and our nonmedical psychological colleagues on the
other. The psychoanalyst must be the primary physician who,
in cooperation with the patient, decides on treatment options
and the appropriateness of consultations and medications.

It follows that the psychoanalyst must be a well-trained physician who is not only versed in the psychotherapy of the neuroses, but also has maintained an active interest in, and study of,
medical problems and complications found in the diagnosis and
treatment of the physical aspects of psychosomatic disorders.
The analyst has to be well acquainted with the benefits and
drawbacks connected with the use of any medications, as well
as the possible dangers and complications associated with the
use of such drugs. He has to be aware of the signs and symptoms that may indicate or anticipate a serious exacerbation of
the patient's illness.

While all of the above are necessary components of the work
of the primary physician, the psychoanalyst, I want to make
clear that it does not negate the need for the services of an
internist and/or surgeon in consultation. Both the patient and
psychoanalytic physician should be aware of the importance of
competent consultation, medical evaluation, investigatory procedures, and laboratory studies. It is often of value to the psychoanalyst to participate in occasional discussions with other
appropriate specialists. The patient should always be informed
of these communications and the reasons for their occurrence.

The consultant, on the other hand, must have an understanding of the psychoanalytic process and be willing to function in an auxiliary advisory role, not directly involved in treatment decisions and instructions. Patients must be allowed to recognize, become more aware of, and analyze how they want to utilize their symptoms for masochistic and provocative needs in the context of the transference. Patients must never be in the position of feeling that they can intimidate one physician in order to exclude the other, especially because the intimidation usually involves a masochistic increase in the level of symptomatology.

The importance of the analyst's therapeutic posture cannot be overemphasized. *If any attempt is made to split the transference with the often-used deceit that the analyst will take care of the emotional problems while the internist takes care of the medical problems, the trio is faced with what it started with—an irreparably split transference that is uninterpretable, and physical symptoms that are unanalyzable.*

There is a related and very important aspect to this split transference. In our experience it is often possible to reduce the medications very early as the patient's physical symptoms improve. It is now essential that the primary physician be able to interpret the longing for the placebo effect of the medications, even those active drugs which may physiologically provide temporary amelioration of the symptoms. Although affects of deprivation and rage—unconscious, denied, or admitted—can at such times be tremendous, in this situation one can interpret dreams and fantasies of the incorporation of the primary object—most often the ambivalently cathected part object. However, early in treatment most patients will deny or fear verbalizing such fantasies, as I pointed out in my discussion of "alexithymia." They often feel that this material is not only shameful and irrelevant but "crazy."

Such transference wishes and manipulations are interpretable only when a cooperative consultant is willing to remain in the background. It is often a fine line to follow. The consultant must not get disturbed when the passively angry patient begins to test the psychoanalytic physician with a mild exacerbation of symptoms. On the other hand, the prescribing or withholding psychoanalyst must have the clinical acumen to evaluate the patient's physiological state and to recognize the dangers of too early withdrawal of medication or the possibility of overmedication.

In all of this the psychoanalyst must repeatedly make clear to the analysand that the patient is in control of the gut and that any medication is used only to ameliorate symptoms; it is not reparative or curative.

The primary physician, the psychoanalyst, must be in a position to explore and interpret all developing activity, whether in the realm of the psyche or the physical. The simultaneous nature of the two activities should be clear and distinct and should be made clear to the patient.

MODIFICATIONS OF TECHNIQUE

If I decide on treatment I tell the patient so and begin treatment as a specific event. As in any unmodified psychoanalysis, I make no promises, but I do indicate in one way or another that there is no reason that the problems cannot be worked through, and if they are, one can expect an amelioration of symptoms. I may give more attention to making this statement than I would in a traditional psychoanalysis. However, I do my best to indicate that the understanding of the conflicts and associations are the responsibility of the patient.

It is here that added parameters or psychotherapeutic maneuvers must be considered. If the patient is in massive denial, as I illustrated in one of my clinical vignettes, a certain education of the observing self may be necessary. Usually in these early stages of treatment the analyst cannot sit back and expect the patient to take the initiative in free association. There are some exceptions as will be demonstrated in the second clinical example described below.

One must often remind patients that their symptoms occur at times when other people might feel hurt or angry. It is important to stress that the patients are afraid of their feelings and prone to shame or even devastating humiliation over any loss of control over them.

INTERPRETATIONS

I want to emphasize how crucial it is to interpret the defenses of these patients early in treatment, rather than call immediate attention to aggressive or sexual wishes and impulses.

Phallic and oedipal concerns should be left for the development of a triadic transference (the more traditional transference neurosis). If these concerns appear early, of course, they must be addressed. When sexual associations erupt in the transference early in treatment they may be primitive in origin. They often are an attempt to control, and do not represent any conscious sexual interest in, the analyst (Hogan, 1983c, pp. 134–137; 1983d, p. 158). After all, an attempt at seduction need not be indicative of sexual interest or even erotic feeling.

I direct specific attention to the punishing superego, which I verbalize simply as "conscience." If possible I interpret the intensity of feelings of shame. In some cases this is again an educative endeavor in which one illustrates the avoidance of feeling because of the (presumed or interpreted) sense of humiliation.

With appropriate but unchallenging comments and interpretations the psychoanalyst illustrates the patient's intolerance of aggressive and libidinal impulses. Self-punishment and potentially suicidal activities are pointed out in these early weeks of treatment (Hogan, 1983d, 1989, 1990). The need for control and the fear of loss of control are repeated themes for interpretation when they are verbalized or behaviorally expressed by the patient; many patients withhold verbalization until they understand their denial. Interpretation must be careful to avoid any possibility of precipitating a sense of humiliation. The analyst is always mindful of the simultaneity of behavior and conscious or unconscious subjective states, and communicates this directly or indirectly to the patient.

In the initial phase of treatment patients are exquisitely sensitive to any observations that they can possibly interpret as contemptuous, accusations of childishness, or indications of some loss of control.

When anxiety arises or consciousness of conflict develops, reassurance is not only of no help, but may assist the patient to return to denial. As anxious as these patients may become, it is destructive to imitate the reassuring parent. One does well to remember Boyer's observation (1980) that "the best substitute parenting one can afford the patient is to hew as closely as possible to the classical analytic model" (p. 206). Utilizing some modifications or parameters early in treatment does not mean indulgence or supportive measures.

The analyst can point out some relevant aspects of psychic reality. One of the reasons these patients are so fearful of acknowledging their wishes and fantasies is their unconscious and conscious fear of acting on their impulses. This naturally leads to their need for illusory control of self and object. Whenever fear of action appears in associations, it is easily interpretable. The psychoanalyst often may proceed to generalize that a fantasy or wish differs from action. When appropriate, the analyst may also comment that one does not have to act on a wish if it is not to one's benefit to do so. I trust that any psychoanalyst recognizes that this interpretation must be given time and time again in a variety of contexts with a multitude of changes in vocabulary: it takes time for patients to recognize that they are dealing with a primitive wish and not an uninhibitable impulse.

This bit of psychic reality is intimately related to another ubiquitous and threatening unconscious conflict: defense against the need for immediate gratification (and action). Examples of this conflict are usually interpretable early in treatment if the psychoanalyst is wary of saying anything that the patient might translate as shameful. If patients feel accused of being inordinately demanding or greedy they often retreat to a protective period of denial ("alexithymia") that prolongs the psychoanalytic process. Patients with pregenital regressions will have to discover as soon as is tolerable that primitive demands for immediate gratification (their unconscious greediness) are really fundamental problems in their illness. As time progresses it is hoped that patients will be able to take a less judgmental and contemptuous attitude toward themselves and their impulses. The sadistic superego will have been examined and the introjects illuminated as demons from the past rather than present-day persecutors.

Minor Modifications: Time

If I decide to see the patient in what I hope will eventually result in successful psychoanalytic treatment, I institute the usual four- or five-times-per-week psychoanalytic schedule. I am extremely careful in my questioning and my interpretation of a patient's breaks in the schedule, as one should always be with a psychoanalytic patient.

There will always be patients who for one reason or another cannot afford the time or cannot participate in an analytic experience. These patients I handle in the conventional manner of instituting brief psychoanalytically oriented psychotherapy on a two- or three-session-per-week schedule.

Minor Modifications: The Use of the Couch

In seminars and in group discussions with psychoanalysts who work with psychosomatic patients the question frequently arises as to whether it is better to see these individuals *vis-à-vis* than to place them on the couch. Some of my colleagues feel that the more severely disturbed patients should be treated *vis-à-vis*. Others seem to feel that any psychosomatic patient is regressed enough that very destructive and chaotic transference reactions (or defenses against them) can occur when the patient is on the couch, holding that it is important to aid the patient's reality testing by maintaining a *vis-à-vis* posture.

I have respect for these opinions and the analysts who propose them. However, I am inclined to place any person in psychoanalysis or intensive psychoanalytic psychotherapy (four or five times per week) on the couch unless the patient objects strongly. I have observed that the patient's reaction to the separation can be valuable and interpretable. I also feel that any refusal to lie on the couch is loaded with potentially analyzable conflict.

Patients in brief psychoanalytically oriented psychotherapy are treated *vis-à-vis*.

CLINICAL ILLUSTRATIONS

Case 1: A young man was ostensibly cooperative and communicative in a rather formal and detached manner. He seemed capable only of a shallow presentation of his fantasy life. A paucity of dreams accompanied his obvious reluctance to verbalize feelings. Early in treatment, if occasionally I had some contributing information from an infrequent dream or unrecognized fantasy, he might allow as how he had some emotional reaction to psychoanalysis. Less often, he might even acknowledge some annoyance at treatment, but not at the analyst. I was dealing with the condition of denial at times labeled alexithymia.

Although some of the minor modifications mentioned above were instituted, it was the handling of an external life experience that precipitated a profound change in the clinical picture. The patient's father died, and as is my practice, I charged for the two accompanying missed treatment sessions. The patient's narcissistic hurt and rage were immense. He sought consultations with other professionals. At least one psychiatrist agreed with him about his unfeeling physician and recommended a change of therapists.

He did not follow the advice to terminate treatment with me. Despite his rage he reluctantly continued with the psychoanalytic process. His slowly improving but episodic attacks of colitis went into complete remission for some months. Now that he felt justified and free of doubts and shame he began to verbalize the hostility that he had consciously felt and denied over the previous period of treatment. He reviewed every real and fantasied neglect or slight that he had experienced since his first day of therapy. Each new remembrance seemed to further support and justify his judgments of my coldness and incompetence (see the discussion of suppression, denial, and projective mechanisms in chapter 9). The denial and splitting with associated mechanisms occasioned by his primitive superego and superego precursors became an understandable subject for analysis. His primitive but rich fantasy life was available for psychoanalytic work. The treatment proceeded over a relatively short time span to a resolution of physical symptoms, but over a much longer period to the resolution of the accompanying emotional conflicts.

In cases such as this, the resolution of defenses can be dramatic and not infrequently related to an external event. This patient's defensive mechanisms are not always characteristic of inflammatory bowel disease patients and the dramatic change is not a universal experience. When it does occur it is a response made possible by the preparatory work described above. One of the most interesting features in this case is how the real psychoanalysis began with the verbalization of a hostile response to a presumed injury.

On the surface, one would not consider this a positive transference. It is true that our recognition of the complexities of transference has widened since Freud's early discoveries. In Freud's description of the beginning of a psychoanalysis (1913b, p. 139) he observed that the emergence of a positive transference was necessary for the work to progress. If this is true, how in my case did the patient's verbalization of extreme rage herald the beginning of a positive (workable) transference? I believe that, first, there was the newfound trust that had evolved from his experience with the constancy and honesty of the analyst. Second, my previous interpretations of his overbearing conscience (sadistic superego) had helped give him permission for the expression of feeling. Third, he had what he experienced as an outside reality to buttress his response to the projections of judgment—which he in part had recognized as his own construction.

To abstract a bit, in effect this patient for the first time separated his perceptions of the psychoanalyst from his experience with the punishing introjected fragments of primitive perceptions of the primary object. His willingness to finally accept that my charge for the sessions was a matter of personal interest and not a punitive deprivation allowed him some freedom of expression. He did not enjoy compromising his feeling of entitlement (Murray, 1964) but he gained a greater recognition of reality.

His incorporated superego demons had continually attacked his wishes and impulses with their own sadistic contempt. His lapses in control, his presumed childish verbalizations, the assumed pratfalls he subjectively judged when he attempted to assert himself, had all been material for his mocking internal dialogue. I do not think that we should be surprised to recognize that such newfound freedom from subjectively experienced demons might occasion a positive response, even though cloaked in a cover of rage.

This type of massive denial and attempts at control are not unusual in psychosomatic patients. The extent of the denial may be correlated with the severity of psychosomatic symptomatology, but this is certainly not always the case. I think that the following case demonstrates that many people with inflammatory gut disease utilize defensive maneuvers other than massive denial in the initial phases of treatment.

Case 2: This patient's symptoms were as serious and life-threatening as those of any whom I have successfully treated. This clinical vignette illustrates how an emergency may be handled without endangering the patient's welfare or compromising a future psychoanalytic position.

A young man had a history of Crohn's disease of the colon and the rectum for the previous seven years, and was suffering from a severe relapse of six months' duration. He had had multiple hospitalizations for bleeding, bacteremia, and other crises, with repeated attempts at hyperalimentation and pre-scriptions of every conceivable medication.

The most recent exacerbation had included one additional hospitalization. Despite the complications associated with sur-gery in Crohn's disease, colectomy had been recommended. His parents had been told that he would die if there was no surgical intervention. When I saw him he was severely emaci-ated and unable to walk without help.

I obtained a preliminary history and knowledge of the labo-ratory findings as well as some information in his physician's report and recommendations, before the consultation. At a later date I obtained, with his permission, copies of the hospital summaries. The patient and his parents desperately wanted to avoid surgery, and psychoanalytic treatment was a last resort.

I had no choice but to use the couch. He could not sit. I did not separate out the early sessions for an investigative phase to evaluate the situation as was recommended above.

I did contact a cooperative internist for future consultation who could make arrangements for hospitalization, should we deem that necessary.

I told the patient that I saw no reason that he could not handle these problems and that I thought I could be of help. I was quite clear about the obvious—there was no promise or guarantee, but we were going to try. I emphasized that what we were trying to do depended upon him and his work. I also acknowledged the real possibility that we might find it necessary to interrupt treatment for a surgical intervention.

The patient revealed that he had very little hope of any help from psychiatric treatment. He had been subjected to past attempts at supportive therapy, an expression of skepticism indicating a degree of spontaneous honesty not always observed in the early treatment of psychosomatic patients. His open dis-agreement represented some tolerance for his own doubts and hostilities. He was quite verbal, and unlike case 1, he was well aware of his severe emotional conflicts. Within the first week of treatment he led me back to some of the problems that he recognized had preceded the current exacerbation of his physical illness.

The patient was quite conscious of the ruminations that troubled and frightened him. One major difficulty was that no physician either listened to or asked him to talk about his feelings and anxieties. My colleagues and I have found that such a state of affairs is not uncommon in psychosomatic patients who have been treated surgically or pharmaceutically. It is extremely important to give any patient not only ample but extended time to talk during the investigative interviews. This may seem frustrating to the physician who is dealing with a patient engaged in massive denial as was case 1, but it is good medicine, nevertheless.

He was concerned with what he felt had been a series of humiliating experiences at the hands of a former friend. He was afraid of his violent fantasies about this individual, and was afraid that he might act on them. As he opened up verbally he discovered brutally sadistic fantasies that he had not even been aware of concerning this past friendship. Ultimately, his past masochistic adaptation to life was correlated with sadistic and masochistic wishes.

Just a few months after entering treatment, he was driving himself to his sessions. Within the year he was gainfully employed for the first time in years.

I trust that I have clarified some of the major modifications that some colleagues and I have found helpful in the initiation of psychoanalytic treatment of these patients. I am not sure whether this early work should be called "psychoanalytic psychotherapy" or "preparatory psychotherapy," but I believe that definitions are relatively unimportant if the stance is a nonreassuring psychoanalytic one, and if the ultimate work evolves into psychoanalysis with a clearly analyzable transference neurosis.

Chapter 15
Transference

In this volume there are repeated references to, and descriptions of, individual transference problems in the discussion of clinical material, some of which will be reviewed below, where my emphasis is on the special qualities of the transference reactions of colitis patients.

If a patient makes notable use of pregenital defenses, psychoanalysts often divide the transference into two areas: narcissistic transference and transference neurosis. We shall see that this clear line of division, although useful and historically important, is a bit too sharp if one is looking for a reasonably accurate description of the clinical findings.

What is of greater significance is the analysis of dyadic (pregenital) defenses early in the treatment before proceeding to the delineation of the primitive drives. In the early phases of treatment spontaneity and free association are impossible for the individual who suffers the physical effects of inflammatory disease of the colon. When pregenital defenses are analyzed we see the emergence of greater spontaneity, the rich fantasy life of the patient, and triadic concerns. This is the traditional transference neurosis with its phallic and oedipal content. We must not forget that in all patients fluctuations between dyadic and triadic associations occur throughout the psychoanalysis or psychoanalytic psychotherapy.

There are specific qualities in the transference analysis of patients with colitis that differ from those of other patients. Like those with other narcissistic disorders they defend themselves from phallic and oedipal conflict with archaic dyadic mechanisms. But an interesting personality quality—to me so far indefinable—often allows one to make a tentative diagnosis before the patient voices a complaint, a quality reflected during the early observations of transference in the wary, withdrawn nature of these patients' presentation of themselves. This characteristic of their communications is not apparent in the discussion of transference below, but it is distinct in those individuals who suffer from inflammatory disease of the bowel. It may be attributed to a greater use of denial and a more obsessive suppression of affect than is commonly observed in other patients who display psychosomatic symptoms.

Freud introduced the concept of transference in *Studies on Hysteria* (Breuer and Freud, 1893–1895), and made detailed discussion of the phenomenon in the "Dora" case (1905). The "Fragment of an Analysis of a Case of Hysteria" is a particularly appropriate place to begin a presentation of the problems in the transference in patients with psychosomatic disorders. (Although we are specifically discussing problems in the transference treatment of inflammatory disease of the gut, such concerns are often shared by other psychosomatic patients.) This patient of Freud's, with her cough, her migraine headaches, and her self-destructive transference relationship, introduces us to the difficult, but analyzable, transference reactions of the psychosomatic patient.

In his discussion of Dora's negative transference Freud asked:

> If cruel impulses and revengeful motives, which have already been used in the patient's ordinary life for maintaining her symptoms, become transferred on to the physician during treatment, before he has had time to detach them from himself. . . . [H]ow could the patient take a more effective revenge than by demonstrating upon her own person the helplessness and incapacity of the physician? [1905, p. 120].

Here Freud introduces us to his patient who insisted on demonstrating his perceived incapacities by her termination of treatment. One could note that in our contemporary treatment of psychosomatic patients they too may sometimes terminate. However, one also sees that such patients take milder revenge with self-destructive manipulations in their exacerbation of symptoms, or, later in the analysis, self-destructive acting out.

My psychoanalytic colleagues and I (see Acknowledgments) often discuss one of the most important characteristics of the psychosomatic transference: *Psychosomatic patients very seldom demonstrate their somatic symptoms during treatment sessions. When they do, it is an acute, important unverbalized presentation of a negative transference* that must be explored, understood, and verbalized by the patient and the physician.

In the Dora case, Freud demonstrated by implication the sadistic impulses and self-destructive masochistic utilization of their derivatives that we now associate with all pregenital regressive defenses like those shown by psychosomatic patients. Freud anticipated the contradictions inherent in handling specific impulses to harm, humiliate, or destroy the primary object or the transference object.

UNIVERSALITY OF TRANSFERENCE

Freud (1925, p. 42) observed the ubiquity of transference and described how it arises spontaneously in all human relationships. There seems to be general agreement among psychoanalysts today that transference occurs in every association between members of the human species (Freud, 1909, 1925; Greenacre, 1954; Bird, 1972; Brenner, 1976; Gill and Muslin, 1976).

Despite the general agreement on the universality of the phenomenon there are a number of psychoanalysts who feel that they can distinguish between outside reality and the subjective perception of reality in the transference. These authors are willing to define the difference between the transference relationship and the real relationship with the patient, a distinction applying an assumption that the psychoanalyst is the ultimate authority on what is "real" and what is "transference." I find any such certainty of definition difficult to justify empirically, logically, or linguistically.

Some of these investigators feel that transference must be "maintained" or "developed" or they see it only as a product of the psychoanalytic relationship. It is true that transference is most commonly defined in the context of psychoanalysis, but it is interesting that Bird (1972) was so impressed with the universality of the phenomenon in all human relationships that he made a very apt contribution to psychoanalytic definition: ". . . transference would seem to me to assume characteristics of a major ego function" (p. 267). I (Hogan, 1983c, 1992) agree with Bird. The ego transfers its past experiences into every human relationship. The more general and ubiquitous transferences commonly represent the more primitive experiences.

In 1969 Loewenstein discussed the attempts of a variety of authors (Sterba, 1934; Zetzel, 1956; Greenson, 1965; Greenson and Wexler, 1969) to narrow or widen the concept of transference. Greenson (1971) attempted to further justify his limitations on the concept and to separate out the concept of a "realistic" working relationship between analyst and patient. Sandler, Dare, and Holder (1973) presented a further discussion of the problem.

Without belaboring this early history further, I restate my earlier positions (1983c) when I noted my substantial agreement with the condensation by Gill and Muslin (1976):

> Freud accepted the existence of a personal relationship with the patient as a necessary and inevitable part of the analytic set-up, in no sense inappropriate, and not to be dealt with as a matter of technique. Though Freud called this relationship "unobjectionable positive transference," or "rapport," many analysts seem to have forgotten that Freud referred to this aspect of the relation with the patient as part of the transference. It now goes by a number of other names—"basic transference" (Greenacre, 1954), "mature transference" (Stone, 1967)—or else is subsumed by more complex concepts—"therapeutic alliance" (Zetzel, 1956), "working alliance" (Greenson, 1965), "real relationship"

(Greenson, 1971), and "the nontransference relationship" (Greenson and Wexler, 1969) [p. 781].

As Gill and Muslin indicate, any attempt to separate the transference to the physician from another type of relationship or from "reality" is definitionally and historically an error. This distinction is important to psychoanalytic theory and of fundamental significance to the success of psychoanalytic treatment.

Every aspect of any patient's cognition of, or feeling about, his or her perception of the analyst should be considered a part of the transference and potentially analyzable. Transference does not appear in fragmented moments of time. In a self-destructive patient, what appears to be the most cooperative positive transference (and could be viewed by some as a realistic working alliance) may evolve as analysis progresses into a representation of masochistic submission and primitive identification. The psychoanalyst is working with a constantly fluctuating hierarchy of dynamic postures and presentations. What the patient may correctly accept as cooperation today, he may experience as humiliating capitulation tomorrow. What the psychoanalyst and the patient may agree upon as real at one time can at a later date turn out to be a sophisticated reenactment of an infantile experience.

Any attempt to classify a presumably defined part of the relationship as other than transference and call it "working alliance" or "therapeutic alliance" unnecessarily limits the universality of transference. The "working alliance," "real relationship," and so on are all manifestations of the positive transference and do not exist outside of the therapeutic relationship.

Now it might be argued—if we were to use these terms in a purely descriptive way only to describe aspects of positive transference—that their use might be acceptable. We know, however, that the psychoanalysts who originated them meant to describe doctor-patient relationships outside the transference.

Brenner (1979b) observed: "Examination of the clinical evidence offered by proponents for the concepts of therapeutic and working alliance leads the author to conclude that neither concept is justifiable. Both refer to aspects of the transference that neither deserve a special name nor require special treatment" (p. 156).

I agree with Brenner that one should forget such considerations since they only confuse the conceptual model and contaminate Freud's "positive transference" with nonanalytic terms. At best modification of terms suggests that there is an area of the analysand's personal experience with an analyst that is unavailable for potential analysis. At worst, it would do what the various authors intended: declare an area off-limits for psychoanalysis.

Schwaber (1990) presents an interesting dimension to the discussion:

> It has been my central argument that an interpretative effort which has as its goal to help the patient recognize such a differentiation (between the "real" nature of the analyst and the past internal object), of the truth of which the analyst implicitly has antecedent knowledge, derives from an outlook on reality which can serve to foreclose, rather than to further psychoanalytic inquiry. It is an outlook profoundly different from one which first must pose a question for which the analyst does not yet know the answer: how might the two objects—the one of the past and that of the present, the one within and that without—be logically seen, not as distinct, but as alike? And, as corollary, what might it mean to another even to ask this question? [p. 230].

I should add that in the treatment of the traditional psychoneuroses both patient and physician may share the illusion that they can separate the real or working relationship from the transference relationship and not interfere materially with the psychoanalysis. In the treatment of a patient with bowel inflammation participation in a mutual deceit can be extremely destructive to the analysis of character defenses. If one accepts the apparently cooperative denial as a working relationship there is no possibility of getting past the patient's defensive position.

I trust that I have made my own position clear. To postulate any limitations on the concept of transference as the interpretable defined relationship between psychoanalyst and patient is to commit a grave error historically and definitionally. Even more important, it is an error that profoundly compromises therapy, particularly when treating characterological psychopathology. The mutual understanding between patient and psychoanalyst of the transference in all of its recognizable dimensions is the most important therapeutic tool of psychoanalysis.

As noted elsewhere in this work, only through the understanding of their transference reactions and manipulations are patients with inflammatory colitis able to comprehend their defensive attempts to manipulate the perceived surrounding world. While this recognition is particularly important for all patients with pregenitally defensive postures, it is also relevant to the working through of the more traditional psychoneuroses—disturbances that do not include severe psychosomatic symptoms.

HIERARCHY OF LEVELS OF REGRESSION

I have already called attention to various viewpoints as to what the concept of transference includes and what constitutes a transference neurosis. These differentiations have further complications when one examines the therapeutic relevance of a transference psychosis. Traditionally, transference neurosis is sharply differentiated from varieties of narcissistic transference. Historically, a psychotic transference reaction would have been totally excluded from any discussion of the transference neurosis.

Giovacchini (1975), who has done distinguished work with regressed patients, contributed an intelligent observation on the relativity of these matters:

It is useful to view the object relationship qualities of transference from the viewpoint of an hierarchical continuum. Insofar as any transference is a recapitulation of an infantile state, the types of object relationships typical of such states would be similarly infantile. From this viewpoint, the regression of narcissistically fixated patients would be characterized by primitive object relationships, which are fragmented ones, but in which contact with another person is still possible. . . . Every transference, even those of highly structured psychoneurotics, has a narcissistic element and the converse would also be true [p. 11].

Giovacchini's continuum of regressive positions seems to be consistent with the propositions of Arlow and Brenner (1964, 1969, 1970). However, a relative approach will probably not satisfy a large number of psychoanalysts when it comes to the traditionally accepted, mutually exclusive definitions of the transference with primitive narcissistic features as opposed to the classical concept of the transference neurosis. As a matter of fact a reader might notice that I often refer to the transference neurosis as though it were separate from the more regressive manifestations of transference.

In both the structured psychoneurotic and the more regressed patient with severe psychosomatic symptoms, there are fluctuations in the transference between the reconstitutions of primitive dyadic and more mature triadic relationships of the past. With either the traditional structured psychoneurotic or the psychosomatic patient, we should first deal with narcissistic characterological phases. With the patient who presents us with symptoms of gut inflammation, this approach is of particular importance.

Giovacchini (1979a) reminds us: "Freud did not state that the transference neurosis is derived exclusively from an oedipal conflict. Rather, he emphasized that the transference neurosis encompasses the patient's total psychopathology . . . he made the oedipus complex the central conflictual core, but when dealing with the transference neuroses specifically, he included other primitive psychic elements" (p. 457). Giovacchini describes the essence of analytic transference as "the projection of infantile, or relatively infantile, elements into the mental representation of therapist." He concluded that "The basic

mechanism of all transference is primitive; its content may involve different levels of ego integration" (p. 468).

The analyst must be aware of the patient's state of regression and the particular developmental level of the self and object representational projections (Boyer and Giovacchini, 1980;
Kernberg, 1975, 1976; Giovacchini, 1975, 1979b). Blum (1977)
correctly informs us that "In addition to conflict and defense,
reconstruction now includes archaic ego states and object relations, reaction patterns and developmental consequences" (p.
758). He adds that "though an oedipal transference neurosis
is central to analytic work, depending upon the personality
structure and depth of regression, varying in duration and intensity of preoedipal transference may be discerned or inferred" (p. 781).

It is apparent that some agreement exists among the psychoanalysts mentioned that the transference is a phenomenon
characterized by its mobility as it shifts between developmental
levels. There is less acknowledgment of the need to direct attention to the form as well as the content of the narcissistic elements of this dynamically fluctuating transference. The analyst
should call nonthreatening attention to splitting, obvious denial, and obvious contradiction whenever possible. Again, with
some exception, the analysis of phallic and oedipal conflicts
remains a feature of the later phases of the treatment.

DEPTH OF TRANSFERENCE REGRESSION

I have mentioned elsewhere in this volume (chapter 14) that
"conventional psychoanalytic wisdom teaches us that treatment
and its modifications are dictated by the nature of the underlying neurosis or psychosis regardless of the symptom" (p. 177).
I have also noted that with inflammatory bowel disease we are
seldom able to draw any firm diagnostic impressions as to the
underlying neuroses at the time of our first interview with the
patient. Our experience gives us a clear idea of the patient's
rather primitive characterological defensive position, but it is

impossible to assign a diagnostic category such as hysterical, obsessional, or depressive; or even to clearly differentiate between neurotic, borderline, or potentially psychotic categories.

Some patients display denial to such a degree that an entire hierarchy of emotional conflicts ranging from severe pregenital difficulties to doubts about sexual identity and serious oedipal concerns may be hidden and subsumed by subjective representation of the organic syndrome. It is also a matter of interest that once the archaic defenses are worked through to the point that the organic symptomatology is temporarily or permanently relinquished, the accompanying neurotic structure makes its appearance. In my patients, the major vehicle for this has been the transference. In chapter 14 I detailed the dramatic nature of some early transference reactions, in which occasionally we see a regressive paranoid component. In chapter 12 I called attention to the high incidence of transference psychoses that various psychoanalysts have reported—quite often in patients who were ultimately successfully treated. It is apparent that this regression need not be permanent and does not necessarily compromise transference interpretation.

Giovacchini (1977) shed some light on this state of affairs when he described a patient of his with a narcissistic character disorder: "This situation is different from a masochistic adjustment that is designed to effect a psychodynamic balance; the defensive constellation of my patient was vital to maintaining a total ego coherence instead of dealing with discrete conflicting disruptive impulses" (p. 10). In this vein, we can see that the patient with an inflamed gut can utilize a psychosomatic symptom to maintain what we observe as a parallel denial of serious primitive subjective conflicts, the maintenance of a total ego coherence. That such denial and conflicts may infrequently involve a temporary psychotic regression should not be surprising.

The primitive material that we are working with in the transference involves the projection of the internalized fragmented representations of archaic part objects. They invariably are representations of parts of the perceived primary object in the dyadic transference, even though the parent or surrogate of either gender may be superimposed. This is important to recognize, inasmuch as we are dealing with a struggle between primitive impulses and fragmented precursors of the superego. If one assumes that the gender of the projection reflects historic reality, and indicates an intact superego and the accompanying triadic nature of the projected conflict, it is easy to interpret the impulse and expect an ego integration of the conflict, a response to an oedipal interpretation not unusual in patients with neurotic concerns. In the early work with psychosomatic patients who present an archaic defensive position directly representing ambivalent conflicts with the representation of the primary object, there is little possibility of an integrative ego response. Subjectively, the patient experiences a revengeful, humiliating, and potentially destroying conscience. This "hanging judge" of a conscience bars any acknowledgment of impulses, whether oedipal or preoedipal. The premature interpretation of an impulse will produce one or another defensive response. Analysands in this bind tend to retreat and deny any feeling. Sometimes they terminate analytic treatment and run from the entire area of conflict, the psychoanalysis.

As analytic psychotherapy progresses, it often becomes apparent that avoidance of feeling is not always unconscious, but denied with rationalizing projections. A young woman patient of mine, as she dispensed with her bouts of colitis, for the first time could consciously verbalize her refusal to put her associations into words. It was too terribly "embarrassing." She felt I would find her "too childish," "too crazy," or that she would be "unendurably humiliated." Stubborn refusal to associate is a common phenomenon. When it occurs, the analyst should be grateful if the patient is at least verbalizing conflict over talking about feeling rather than avoiding the entire subject. Some psychoanalysts might communicate a countertransference annoyance at what appears to be stubborn defiance of the analytic rule of free association; whether stated or not, the analyst's stance puts an end to the patient's verbalization of conflict.

Conscious suppression is often revealed in a more dramatic fashion with an apparent transference crisis. In one instance (see chapter 14), a male patient's narcissism was wounded severely when I charged for time that he missed on the occasion of his father's death. He responded with rage and reviewed the previous months of therapy, listing all of my real or imagined defects as well as all of the indignities that he felt he had suffered at my hands since the beginning of treatment. In this case, as in some others, the patient had denied, over a long period of time, most of his personal feelings for, as well as any aggressive feelings toward me, despite repeated questions and interpretative suggestions.

The above two examples are typical of the transferences in colitis patients, but in most cases the responses are not as reasonable as the conscious admissions of the young woman who nevertheless had engaged in a prolonged period of denial with accompanying psychosomatic symptoms. Even after working through some of her intense feelings of humiliation there were long phases in which her mild paranoid projections indicated her absolute conviction of my humiliating and destructive judgments. Like the young man above, she had gone through intervals of denying and suppressing her associations without informing the analyst.

Treatment involves the slow process of working out the projection of judgments, then the projective identifications, and, later, the projection of impulses. One can easily visualize some of the problems with countertransference, of which I provide details in chapter 16.

The fundamental unconscious problem in patients with inflammatory colitis is the intensity of primitive sadistic aggression in the ambivalence toward the primary object. These patients have been forced in infancy to utilize the archaic defense of denial, resting as it often does on splitting and fragmentation with paranoid mechanisms. Just as the primitive controlling aggression is denied, so is the accompanying infantile need for immediate gratification and action.

In order to maintain their denial, patients must fantasy complete control of their impulses and their perceptions of the object, using the projective mechanisms mentioned above. Sperling (1961, 1967, 1968, 1978a) noted that these patients used their objects as "fetishes."

The fantasies of omnipotent control of subject and object representations are further reinforced and maintained by the fragmentation and splitting that is so much a part of this regressive defensive picture. The splits (Hogan, 1983b, p. 142) often are clearly definable in terms of self perceptions, object perceptions, self representations, and object representations. There is a continuum between those that are conscious and seem to be under the patient's control and those that are denied and repressed and out of the patient's awareness.

Grotstein (1981) presents us with a similar pattern in his discussion of the general process of psychic splitting. "The act of splitting may be active or experienced as passive, and we can speak of macroscopic and microscopic splitting" (p. 10). He also reminds us that "splitting can be done (a) under the auspices of perceptual or cognitive thinking where discriminations are required; and (b) defensively, which involves counter cathexis against unwanted perceptions and feelings" (p. 78). Grotstein makes the important observation that splits that are experienced as passive lead to a feeling of fragmentation.

This leads us to two important clinical points in our understanding of the transference in patients with inflammatory colitis. First, those splits that seem to be under the patient's control—"active" and apparently "under the auspices of perceptual or cognitive thinking" in Grotstein's terms—are not that much under conscious cognitive control. These splits are usually maintained by rationalizations of a projective, or occasionally paranoid, nature. The more simple and benign expressions include "this is not important, he will not be interested," "this is insulting so why bring it up," "it is not relevant," "he will think I am crazy." In the early stages of treatment rationalizations are so much a part of the patient's psychic equilibrium that he or she does not even realize that material is being withheld. It is all part of the patient's unconscious fantasy of omnipotent control. It is also a posture to which patients can return defensively long after they have recognized the manipulation and have "graduated" to more spontaneous free association. A good example was a young man in his fourth year of psychoanalytic psychotherapy who, whenever he became defensive in the transference, consciously verbally disowned the significance of any associations that did not fit the preconceived point he was "trying to make."

Second, there are few patients who can acknowledge their own passivity. Although it is important to interpret the form and character of demonstrable splitting, denial, and contradiction early, I recommend that discretion be used in the interpretation of the projective rationalizations that maintain the splitting. Splits experienced as passive can lead to a feeling of fragmentation. An indiscreet interpretation of projection can force the patient into a position of recognizing his or her own passivity and lack of control and bring on a sense of fragmentation. The typical response in this case is to withdraw or run.

The subjective world of these individuals allows little freedom for any adult feeling of responsibility that is relatively free of guilt. They are constantly in the hands of the superego's judgmental demons, experienced personally and painfully, as personal antagonists which patients project in every relationship—particularly the one involving psychoanalytic transference. Their world is made up of shoulds with the rewards of shame and guilt for failure.

These patients unconsciously feel that they must have what they want immediately. If they do not get it, a destructive rage to control or destroy ensues, a feeling taboo to an equally destructive superego. Ego integration is severely compromised, and conflict is handled by denial and masochistic self-punishment, with attempts at self-destruction. It is worth emphasizing that the analyst is not dealing with an ego that can recognize a "death wish." One is dealing with an ego that is terrified of an intense, usually unconscious, impulse to humiliate or destroy the beloved object. On an unconscious level the impulse seems to demand immediate satisfaction. It is the recapitulation, and the derivative, of a conflict from early infancy.

Bird (1972) wondered about the vicissitudes of these impulses in the transference:

> [N]egative, destructive tendencies [i]n contrast to libidinal drives [p. 287] . . . run into a good deal of trouble . . . [in being experienced in the transference] ending up at best as wishes, . . . those involving literal destructive acts, seem to stand little chance of entering the transference at all [p. 288]. . . .
> [W]hen a patient behaves violently in his daily life and reports this to us, we may not tell him to stop, we may directly warn him of the consequences [p. 289]. . . .
> [T]he patient's literal attempts to destroy the analyst, probably represent in the transference neurosis, . . . the patient's own attempts to destroy certain aspects of himself, . . . and instead to destroy others [p. 259].

Dynamically, Bird is right. When a patient experiences the impulse to or uncovers the fantasy of attacking the analyst, he is ready to attack his perception of an internalized representation, which has been projected. The introject is a part of the self—an archaic fragment of a primitive superego. Nevertheless, unconsciously and with evolving consciousness, the patient's perception of the analyst (introject) becomes dramatically real and constitutes a tremendous perceived threat to the patient and to the patient–analyst relationship, to say nothing of what is an *apparent* threat to the psychoanalyst. Freud's Dora, it seems, acted out the destruction of the patient–psychoanalyst relationship, and conceivably fantasied the fulfillment of an unconscious or conscious fantasy of Freud's destruction.

Bird (1972) certainly captures the reciprocal nature of the self- and object-directed impulses toward destruction. Sperling (1967, 1968) too emphasized that conflict about primitive aggression plays a determinative part in psychosomatic symptoms. (To be precise, the subjective expression of self-directed aggression, whatever the content of the patient's fantasies about himself may be, is paralleled by his observations of physiological self-destruction—psychosomatic symptoms. It is also paralleled by the patient's experience of the subjective representations of the colonic activity—again psychosomatic symptoms.)

When we speak of aggression in psychoanalytic terms, the subjective feelings always have content—fantasy. The fantasy may be suppressed if action is involved, but when a patient acts out we are analyzing a subjective state: we and the patient are witnessing behavioral activity. The psychoanalyst observes, as does the patient, but the patient also subjectively experiences the impulse to act as well as the mild omnipotent euphoria that parallels the action. An aggressive or masochistic fantasy may also be suppressed if symptoms are involved, in which case the analyst and the patient are witnessing the symptom, the former as an outsider and the latter as a witness to the event as well as a person experiencing a subjective representation of physical and physiological symptomatic activity.

INTERPRETATION OF PRIMITIVE DEFENSIVE POSITIONS

The technical problem in the early interpretative approaches to the transference is the avoidance of interpreting libidinal or aggressive impulses at a time when the patient's ego is still unprepared to deal with them. As long as the patient's outside life and transference life are ruled by primitive fragmented superego precursors, the patient will either deny and retreat into withdrawal or deny and run from treatment. Subjectively, there's just too much humiliation, guilt, and fear. We can, however, deal with this transference problem once colitis patients can observe and acknowledge the judgmental intensity and the self-destructive nature of their own consciences. Early interpretations can be directed toward the patient's guilt, shame, and self-destruction. The suicidal nature of the patient's behavior and symptomatology can be observed or suggested in the beginning phases of psychoanalytic psychotherapy. This type of superego-oriented interpretation is appropriate. It seems to be safer for patients to see themselves as victims of their consciences, than to acknowledge responsibility, with accompanying shame and guilt, for their sexual or sadistic impulses.

In this context, when the material is available, one can highlight the judgmental nature of the patient's transference projections. In some patients who use massive denial and projection such material is not readily available; that is, until an outside situation allows the patient to feel justified in the expression of indignation and rage in the transference.

I discussed above and in chapter 14 (pp. 187–189), the treatment of a patient who responded with intense narcissistic hurt to my charges for missed sessions. This man could feel justified in his rage at such a perceived injustice, yet despite consultive advice to terminate, his unconscious understanding seemed to force him to continue treatment without any insistence on my part. He was able to gain insight into his projections of my hatred, contempt for, and punishment of him. He could begin to distinguish his own punitive conscience, his own persecuting demons of internalized part object representations from his perceptions of me as an analyst who he had to admit, was ostensibly there to help. He regretted relinquishing some of his fantasies of omnipotence and entitlement (J. M. Murray, 1964) but was obtaining a more mature perception of his own independent existence.

I want to be clear here. I am not contrasting a reality, a working alliance, or whatever else with a transference experience. We are merely working within the transference, broadening the transference experience and recognizing *relative* levels of maturity, independence, and spontaneity.

Another patient of mine with a pattern of denial that some might call alexithymic, was able to profit by a transference reaction to an environmental event in my waiting room. He had heard the loud abusive accusations of a paranoid patient, in consultation, penetrating my office door. When he entered my office he described a fantasy of coming in and saving me from a rather bloody attack. As is often demonstrable with colitis patients, despite the apparent integrity of my body, he had little immediate recognition that the scenario he had described was a fantasy. After my interpretation that his subjective drama might represent some angry feelings and fantasies of his own, for the first time he talked albeit superficially about this possibility. He admitted fears of being just such a "maniac," and went on to his frequent fears of being crazy, but added how ashamed he was of his silly fears and preoccupations. In fleshing out my interpretation I suggested that in his fantasies he was the attacker. He denied it but his face paled—a reaction that I called to his attention. That night he had a dream of an affectionate gesture toward me. His rendition the following day was accompanied by shame and humiliation. I superficially interpreted it as a wish for reconciliation and forgiveness, and emphasized the intense shame he felt over such wishes. He went on to volunteer anxiety about possibly being a sissy and later admitted adolescent and early adult fears of being a homosexual. His "alexithymia" was gone. I do not claim that his denial was erased. For some period of time, whenever threatened, he temporarily retreated to massive denial and other control mechanisms. As with most colitis patients, he used denial as a defense throughout treatment.

All of which leads me to a closely allied and somewhat difficult area of transference interpretation. Patients with pregenital defenses try to avoid admitting a want or a need because they want so much, and so intensely. Their unconscious, and, one always hopes, their ultimately perceived, conscious need for *immediate gratification or action* is so great that they carefully anticipate, and try to avoid, any chance of confrontation. They dodge not only the confrontation, but any possibility of verbalizing feelings about it. They feel unable to tolerate the exquisite pain of narcissistic hurt and rage. In the early weeks, months, and even years of analytic treatment, colitis patients are invariably aware of the time in the analytic hour and anticipate the perceived dismissal and abandonment at the end of the session.

It is always helpful if patients can encompass and understand the immediacy of their needs early in treatment. But even the most carefully phrased interpretation can be experienced as an accusation of greediness and childishness, and accompanied by shame and retreat. I have discovered that if an inadvertent opportunity has not presented itself, the analyst can usually call attention to the patient's need to be aware of time and how it helps control the pain of frustration. Again we see that these individuals are willing to see themselves as victims of frustration and pain rather than acknowledge responsibility for what they may experience as childish greediness. As our patients become more and more aware of the pain associated with the feeling of frustration it is not difficult, utilizing specific events, to proceed with gentle interpretations of their needs for immediate gratification.

With the variety of interpretations possible, one repeatedly interprets the patient's need to *control*—almost everything: his or her own conscience, those humiliating and punitive superego fragments, any awareness of impulses, any verbalization of fantasy, the perceptions of the psychoanalyst, and the patient's own perceived reactions to the perceptions. These patients have a desperate desire to control feeling, unaware that one feels first, often accompanied by fantasy and elaboration. They know what they *should* feel. Colitis patients have great difficulty in subjectively acknowledging motivation; it seems too far from conscious control. Yet an acknowledgment and eventual subjective acceptance is necessary. An intellectually acute patient can talk about motivation—even personal motivation—in abstract terms, but for a long time remain unable to acknowledge the personal experience. This is no area for cognitive psychology if one expects a resolution of the physical pathology.

It is fascinating that, despite a need to control thoughts, feelings, and associations, these patients seem to lack control over the gut. Subjectively, they experience their perceptions of intestinal activity as a total lack of control. As has been mentioned so often, the immediate aim of the symptomatic treatment is to allow patients to recognize that they do control those internal representations of intestinal activity and that along with the control of those representations there are corresponding changes in the physical and physiological activity of the colon.

Here, Sperling can briefly contribute some illustrative and instructive material. In her paper on transference (1967) she illustrates that "to feel meant to him that he would have to act on his feelings instantly in reality. In analysis the patient succeeded in convincing himself that he could tolerate awareness of impulses without immediate discharge, as he had done previously in the diarrhea and as he now had the urge to do in reality" (p. 346). She also discusses a nine-year-old boy with ulcerative colitis: "I had to interpret incessantly that I was not his mother and that I knew, and could help him to know, that he could tolerate his impulses consciously without endangering himself or others. . . . he stopped running to the bathroom. . . . would relax and say, 'I stopped it.' This is an essential experience for the psychosomatic patient: to convince himself that he can control his somatic symptoms" (p. 347). In her (1957) discussion of a 39-year-old male patient with ulcerative colitis she notes that it is "of the utmost importance that the patient at all times conceive of the analyst as the person who expects him to control his own impulses and knows that he can do so, knows that he does not *have* to release them instantly in the somatic symptoms or in equivalent behaviour" (p. 344) and in reference to this same patient: "his wish to surrender to anything to avoid the conscious awareness of such urgent impulses and painful feelings" (p. 345).

Sperling (1946, 1955a, 1957, 1960, 1967, 1968, 1969, 1978b) demonstrated that these patients are terrified of their impulses and accompanying sadistic fantasies on one hand and of their masochistic defensive submissiveness on the other. Many attempt to deny every aspect of the conflict and to present a shallow, withdrawn image of superficial reactivity. With or without this superficial but global defense of denial, there is an overwhelming fear of the underlying impulses and fantasies. She (1967) described a patient who "had the costly choice between getting sick or losing control, which equals 'going crazy' "

(p. 345), a complaint often seen in colitis patients—the fear of going "crazy"—which they equate with losing control, or verbalizing their "crazy" fantasies.

And here we again approach that realm so readily questioned by psychiatrists who have not treated colitis patients with psychoanalytic psychotherapy: Are there or are there not fantasies in these patients? And do fantasies play any role in the reversibility of their symptom complexes? "The proof of the pudding" would seem to lie in our clinical findings and our therapeutic results.

To review: the ego, by way of primitive superego precursors, must defend itself against unintegrated archaic impulses, like the untamed infantile need for either immediate gratification, action, or both. Impulses to action are accompanied by equally archaic fantasies of omnipotent control, humiliation, and destruction, unintegrated fantasies unacceptable to the conscious ego. Consequently, the primitive superego, by way of archaic precursors of reaction formation, directs the sadistic humiliation back toward the ego (narcissistic shame). The primitive needs for destruction can be witnessed and followed in the accompanying masochistic behavioral (acting out) and self-destructive physiological (symptomatic) activities. When recognizing the subjective obsolete precursors to reaction formation one can also begin to make sense out of the patient's archaic undifferentiated subjective ego state with its poorly defined differences between self and object.

This state of affairs perpetuates the early fragmented perceptions of self and object, which allows for the reinforcement of projective mechanisms because the borders between the object and the self are so blurred. The ego has sublimated the primitive fantasy of omnipotent control with some minor differentiations. The fantasy now includes fantasied control over all self and object perceptions and actions.

When we consider the fragile defensive pattern of the ego in patients with inflammatory diseases of the colon, it is not difficult to understand the frequency of psychotic transference reactions.

PSYCHOSES AND TRANSFERENCE PSYCHOSES

Attention has elsewhere (chapter 12) been directed to the small number, but extraordinarily high percentage of transference psychoses in this group of patients. A patient of mine gave up her symptomatology (at least temporarily) only to terminate in a paranoid fury directed at me, and other patients had transference projections bordering on paranoid, but in these cases the diagnosis of psychosis depends upon how one defines psychosis. All of this is by way of saying that it is extremely difficult to evaluate reported incidents of transference psychosis in patients who have recovered with treatment. From my own experience and from my review of the literature I conclude that at best we are dealing with a lot of projection and an equal magnitude of projective identification. One handles these transferences carefully. Whether or not one calls the transference reactions "psychotic" may be a choice of terminology.

In general medical literature one often reads of the association between psychosis and inflammatory disease of the large bowel (see chapter 12). There are reports of a number of patients in whom alternating intervals of colonic and psychotic activity were observed. Others have cautioned the unwary to avoid psychiatric treatment or psychoanalysis because of the danger of psychosis attendant upon the intervention. A review of this aspect of the literature is not the immediate concern of this book, but I will make a brief comment. In some ways I am very impressed by the apparent fragility of the defenses in colitis patients. In other ways these troublesome pregenital barriers seem quite stable and protective. I have often observed temporary lapses of reality testing in the transference life of my patients; I have not, however, noted any particular association of colitis with paranoid or psychotic reactions in their past histories. Nor have I observed this association in the histories of patients whom I have seen in consultation or in those whose treatment I have supervised. On the other hand, it is difficult to evaluate the automatic screening that must occur with patients before they decide to consult, or are sent for consultation with, a psychoanalyst.

OEDIPAL TRANSFERENCE

Any patient whose defensive pattern has been marked by denial, isolation, splitting, fragmentation, and projection tends to revert to these defenses whenever psychologically threatened. The tendency to a temporary regressive state seems to be more pronounced in people depending heavily on pregenital defenses than is the case in the more traditional psychoneuroses. In patients who have had psychosomatic symptoms of colonic inflammation denial is a part of the clinical picture at any stage of the psychoanalysis.

As the ego of a patient can progressively integrate defensive regressions into transference and life experience, an apparently more mature stage of development appears. The need for the subjective representations of pain and chaos in the internalized experience of colonic activity is given up. As the patient dispenses with these psychological needs there is an accompanying recovery from the physiological responses—bouts of ulcerative colitis or Crohn's colonic disease.

At the same time a more typical neurotic structure emerges and symptomatic depression and/or phobic responses make an appearance. While phallic and oedipal themes have reverberated through the more archaic material from the beginning of treatment, the ego gains the freedom to understand, take responsibility for, and integrate triadic conflicts of the phallic and oedipal phases of development.

One transferential concern is that, as with most psychosomatic patients, there is a fluctuating period, as the somatic symptoms are given up, when one usually sees oscillating episodes of acting out and of depression. At these times suicidal ideation is a common accompaniment. Naturally, one should remain the analyst—listen and interpret. To sympathize or display anxiety only reduplicates the maternal role and contributes to regressive activity such as the possibility of acting out the patient's fantasies.

I hope and trust that the progression from the cautionary tales about pregenital defenses to the more cheerful review of oedipal neurosis is enough of an indication of treatability of this group of patients. I can also add that in the experience of my immediate colleagues and myself we have seen no severe or prolonged exacerbations of the illness, even in those patients who terminated prematurely and whom we were able to follow. If the transference is handled carefully we find that those primitive defenses, although sometimes frustrating to the psychoanalyst and to the cooperating patient, afford reasonable protection for the subject's psychic integrity.

Chapter 16
Countertransference

In patients with psychosomatic symptoms, the accompanying (parallel) psychopathology is seldom schizophrenic or otherwise psychotic. These patients utilize narcissistic defensive maneuvers like those seen in patients with character pathology. Patients with symptoms of an inflamed gut, asthma, or anorexia nervosa have an additional defensive maneuver in their repertoire: they unconsciously use their lives as weapons. Unlike the suicidal threats (and/or attempts) of a depressed or psychotic patient, the self-destructive threats of the psychosomatic patient are not consciously acknowledged until understood and interpreted by the psychoanalyst. To the untrained and uninitiated therapist, the responsibility for handling such a patient can present a formidable and threatening burden.

Many analysts feel that psychosomatic patients are unsuitable for psychoanalytic psychotherapy because attempts to treat them have been uncomfortably unsuccessful. Some psychoanalysts consciously or unconsciously react to their own subjective defenses against the responses to the psychosomatic patient to the transference encounter. Here one is clearly confronting a problem of countertransference.

I believe this is often a matter of education. Many psychoanalysts who have been told that psychosomatic patients are not suitable candidates for psychoanalytic psychotherapy do not follow the successful treatment of such patients in the literature, nor do they allow themselves to become personally therapeutically involved with such cases. Here it is not exactly a matter of countertransference, it is lack of knowledge of the possibilities of successful treatment.

Other psychoanalysts, while acknowledging the therapeutic effects of psychoanalytic treatment, do not want to get involved with difficult, self-destructive patients whose symptoms could be fatal. I believe a conscious decision does not necessarily constitute a countertransference reaction but is common in choosing one's medical specialty.

To anticipate countertransference problems we must first understand the transference position of patients with colitis. Covered in some detail above (chapter 15), the subject nevertheless deserves a condensed general review here. These patients live in a world where they experience little separation from the internalized representations of the primary object (actually fragmented part objects) of identification. All ambivalence toward that object will be subjectively experienced in their projections on the psychoanalyst. On the one hand the patient has the unconscious demand for immediate gratification and love from the projected fragmented self–object; yet on the other hand the patient wants to control, humiliate, and destroy that same projected object representation. These primitive impulses, and accompanying needs for action, have not matured and been integrated in the unconscious ego as wishes. They are demands and impulses that are still defended against in the most infantile fashion. One might say that the problem for the patient is a rather archaic form of the classical negative transference. The patient is dealing with an unconscious, unwanted primitive impulse to destroy the analyst by destroying the psychoanalytic relationship as Freud (1905, p. 120) described in his review of the Dora case. The defenses against the impulse are always compromise formations that carry with them the attempt to gratify, as well as the attempt to deny, the underlying impulse. The presenting unconscious defenses of these undifferentiated patients include both splitting and projective mechanisms. Some psychoanalysts think that the projective mechanisms maintain the splits. Others see a reverse interaction. I believe that there is no maintenance or causality involved here. The two are parts of the same mental process. Grotstein adds (1981):

All projection is projective identification since projection is unthinkable without (a) identity of self being included in the projection, and (b) an acknowledgment of identification secondarily
with the projection or a disavowal of identification with the projection—the latter of which is a negative identification with the
projection nevertheless [p. 213].

Wilson (1989d) has noted that:

[P]sychosomatic patients project unacceptable aspects of the personality—impulses, self-images, superego introjects—onto other
people, particularly the analyst. . . . These patients attempt to
control objects, including the analyst, by unconsciously inducing
the object to experience the conflicts that developed in the patient as a child in the parental relationship [p. 107].

This identificatory process in which the analyst is often induced to experience feelings parallel to the patient's unconscious feelings, has been discussed by a number of psychoanalysts (Rosenfeld, 1952; Klein, 1955; Sperling, 1955b, 1967;
Bion, 1956; Giovacchini, 1975, 1979a,b; Kernberg, 1975, 1976;
Grinberg, 1979; Grotstein, 1981; Hogan, 1983c,d; Porder,
1987).

Some observers seem to feel that the ability to induce an
identification with the patient can attain almost mystical dimensions. They speak as though patients actually project their feelings onto the analyst. While this may be the patient's fantasy,
it is obviously an unconscious fantasy and not a direct invasion.

The colitis patient unconsciously tries to reverse the roles
of analyst–patient, parent–child, and aggressor–victim in order
to place the psychoanalyst in the guilty defensive position consciously felt by the patient in both childhood and in the transference.

Porder (1987) presented a good and reasonable explanation
of the process and put it in the context of all the stages of
development. I think that he depreciated the importance of
regressive primitive mechanisms of merging and splitting in the
successful or unsuccessful utilization of the defensive position

against the analytic process. This is a defensive process that the psychoanalyst sees used more frequently and more effectively in patients with pregenital regression that in patients with more classical transference psychoneuroses.

Fortunately, doctor and patient both have certain common unconscious characteristics, affects, and even fantasies. In my experience, when a pregenitally regressed patient unconsciously provokes a reaction in me, I not infrequently found my response followed by a "double take" in which I recognized the therapeutic interchange. Such subjective responses on my part have included withdrawal, drowsiness, anger, pity, affection, brief sexual interest, and I suppose a number of other affective states. Occasionally, I and others have experienced brief mental states such as a sense of isolation or moments of confusion. Reflection and inquiry always confirm a provocative wish on the part of the patient and ultimately link wish to infantile child–parent conflicts. I have no doubt that projective identification does exist, and that our patient is capable of inducing an identificatory response in the subjective world of the analyst if the potential for such a response is there. The important point is that the analyst be aware of his or her own responses and fantasies, and be able to frame the patient's provocative, demanding, or pleading associations in a nonaccusatory interpretable context.

As Boyer (1979) reflects:

> Over the years I have come to credit with increasing conviction the roles of projective identification and counter identification in the interactions between regressed patients and their therapists. Accordingly, it is my opinion that when I think or fantasize about some person who is important to the patient, I may be responding to his or her need to have me assume some role or attribute of that person [p. 352].

Boyer also emphasizes another observation that agrees with my own findings: "that which is projected remains to a degree unrepressed and the patient maintains some level of continuing to feel what he seeks to project into the therapist, thereby continuing to be preconsciously aware of what he imagines the therapist to experience" (p. 367).

DENIAL AND WITHDRAWAL

Probably the most troublesome and most obvious provocation occurring early in treatment is denial, with both suppression and repression of fantasy and affect—"alexithymia." Our patients display themselves as reactive robots in order to avoid their judgmental consciences and the perceived judgment of the analyst (projected internalized superego fragments). They are also recapitulating an area of infantile conflict, unconsciously identifying with an internalized parental representation who, in the past, displayed similar denial and withdrawal. This object of the patient's infancy was unable to give adequate affective responses to the child's helpless neediness. The patient tries to force the analyst into a reproduction of lack of parental response or interest, at the same time indicating the patient's own lack of response or interest. Is this maneuver effective? One has only to look at the literature to see the "alexithymic" patients' ability to convince a large body of medical observers that he suffers from some organic deficit. The maneuver can be equally effective in the context of therapy: the patient can force an analyst into repeated episodes of sleep and then can terminate treatment in disguised disgust. The patient is defensively even more successful if he or she convinces the psychoanalyst that treatment should be terminated because the patient is untreatable.

This defense is a direct threat to the therapist's trust in his or her own skills, which, unfortunately, at times is intimately tied to omnipotent fantasies. If the bond between confidence and omnipotence is too strong there is little hope that the physician will survive the therapeutic encounter. Treatment will be terminated for one reason or another.

The defensive maneuver, with or without accompanying preconscious or conscious identifications, requires our patience.

An early move toward interpretation may involve minor educational procedures. If the analyst perceives that obvious feelings are denied he or she can safely suggest their presence. In the early stages of treatment (some call it preparatory treatment) one can even note that the patient seems to be unconventionally rational when others might be enraged. When the material warrants, it is important to interpret the strength of the patient's conscience, and how intolerant that conscience is of any feeling. Whenever the conscious recognition of shame comes into associations, its inhibitory relevance, importance, and intensity have to be underlined. In these early days one can occasionally interpret the identification or the projection, but it must be done in a clearly understandable manner and in a reasonable context. It should not threaten the patient's needed illusion of control.

Some colitis patients display no denial and/or withdrawal when introduced to psychoanalytic psychotherapy. An example of such a cooperative initiate was one of my more severely ill patients (see case 2 in chapter 14). This young man was really waiting and hoping to tell someone of his problems. No professional had listened with any real interest to his spontaneous associations. Though he quite frequently utilized denial, usually with splitting, rationalization, and externalization, throughout the early analysis, there was no period in which he denied fantasies, dreams, or feelings. His conscious fears of his sadistic impulses and fantasies were uppermost in his mind. At this point there was little provocation for a hostile countertransference reaction. There was, however, a certain danger of being seduced by the openness and the availability of the material. He certainly projected an omnipotent idealized identification into his perception of the analyst. In this situation therapists must recognize that they have no immediate revelatory interpretations or omnipotent solutions.

Another patient (case 1 in chapter 14) illustrates the type of denial so often described as alexithymia. In the introductory phases of his psychoanalytic psychotherapy there were seemingly few fantasies, virtually no dreams, and an apparent indifference to suggestions about transference feelings. This defense can induce a number of possible countertransference responses, the commonest of which is diagnosis of "alexithymia" with a rather dim outlook for any intensive psychiatric treatment. The hopeful psychoanalyst, anticipating a successful therapeutic encounter, may find his mind wandering and drowsiness compromising his intuitive faculties. One trusts that the analyst's self-knowledge prevents repeatedly falling asleep. On the other hand one may become overtly angry at the patient's lack of cooperation and associations. This response indicates the analyst's conflict about the patient's transference communications. If the analyst's sense of omnipotence is threatened by the patient's projected indifference, the treatment can be in trouble. One cannot be faulted for experiencing the beginnings of such responses, but if physicians expect to uncover and understand their patients' conflicts, it is important to uncover and understand their own responses to their patients' unconscious provocations. It takes time, but if analysts can "hew closely to the classical analytic model" (Boyer, 1980, p. 351) and maintain an interest in their own mental processes they usually find that the bothersome defenses yield to psychoanalytic understanding.

MASOCHISTIC PROVOCATION: SYMPTOM FORMATION

The masochistic subjective representation of colitis is a compromise formation that is overdetermined. It represents a rebellious lack of anal control and an angry sadistic expulsion of the incorporated object. It represents a painful, bloody self-punishment. It represents illness and a demand for love and care from the object. It represents a way to feel that one is punishing the object as one projects and identifies. It can represent innumerable specific original or accumulated fantasies about all of the above and more, such as birth. It can be used as a tool to manipulate and control the personal environment in general and the transference in particular. Here too, is a compromise formation—all the apparent lack of control is paradoxically a subjective process that is used to control.

I can illustrate the overdetermination, projective identifications, and defensive provocation with a vignette from a patient who was well into analysis, but was still occasionally symptomatic. He surprised me at a late date by asking for my card, claiming that he might become suddenly ill and need me. I admit to a momentary sense of unreality. It was as if I were being kidded. I reflected and realized that although he might be unconsciously making fun of me, he was communicating a serious conflict. I asked him what meaning his request might have because he presumably knew my number or could write it down, and why did he expect an attack anyway? In a petulant, regressed manner he complained that I had no sympathy, and that I really did not care about what happened to him. That weekend he was away from home and had a by then unusual, short but acute exacerbation of his colitis, a great deal of pain and blood over a relatively short time. On the following Monday he came in accusing me of leaving him helpless and unattended and of being an incompetent and heartless physician, accusations, at this stage of analysis, that provoked a momentary feeling of indignation on my part. Fortunately, I recognized my own subjective countertransference response to the entire drama whatever it was. I felt a mixture of annoyance and incredulity. This was too far into the treatment! This patient already had too much insight! Yet I was forced to recognize that my own feelings did not reflect the reality of the patient's short but serious weekend exacerbation of his colitis. Something else must be going on. My patient was unconsciously "setting me up."

While I was sorting out my own mental confusion the patient dropped the whole subject and proceeded to what he felt was a separate train of associations: his mother's careful attendance to the cleanliness of his bed that, in the past, he had regularly soiled, and his father's childish demands upon the mother asking her to account for her whereabouts, which she usually did with notes on the refrigerator. I suggested that he might want me to be both father who worried about mother's whereabouts, and mother who took such interest in his illness and cleaned up after him. Perhaps he was angry that I had been indifferent to his needs. He laughed derisively at the interpretation and insisted on the separation of topics in his associations—demanding a recognition of splits between each chain of associations. He felt that in each communication a conscious intended point was to be made. Having displayed his contempt, he then recalled preschool experiences of his mother giving him her picture whenever she was to be away. After a pause he remembered his feeling of rage at me when I had given him a bill for the month rather than my card. Recalling his thoughts about the intense demanding dependency his parents voiced about each other just before the onset of the exacerbation, he allowed as how he might like me if I were more like them, both in taking care of him and in showing my own vulnerabilities and weaknesses as they did. Besides, he was sure that I wanted to give him my card, but that I was withholding it in order to teach him some ridiculous lesson. When I mentioned that mother had never withheld her picture, he said, with some sadness, "I guess you are right."

Here were multiple projections of both parents as dependent helpless people with whom he identified, as well as projections of their depriving qualities, with which he also identified. The latter identification was acted out in his accusations of my incompetence and his laughing, sarcastic denials of my interpretation. Petulant temporary regression is a not uncommon occurrence in colitis patients, but I have noticed a brief annoyance in myself at what I momentarily experience as a childish dodge. It is not difficult to see that this arrogant defensiveness, when unexplained early in the analysis, could elicit overt annoyance, private judgmental withdrawal, or both on the part of the analyst. It can be subjectively frustrating to physicians if and when they feel that their patients have them over a barrel

because the patients are so ill. If the analyst's response is unconscious, one can expect a decision that the case is untreatable by
psychoanalytic psychotherapy.

In the case under discussion we were far enough into analysis that, despite his insistence on rationalization of intent (really
trying to maintain a split and to fragment his associations into
separate topics), my patient was able to recognize his preconscious projections and demands. I should add that the precipitating reason for the regression was the demand by his parents
that he share in payment for the analysis. Here was the depriving mother, not the mother who gave him her picture and
cleaned up after him. As the sessions went on he recognized
the subjective association of my card with mother's picture, with
mother's care, with father's care for mother, and so on. He
also associated to the subjective connections in my perceived
rejection, his parents' depriving expectations, his envy of his
parents' dependence on each other. He identified with each of
these part objects and their accompanying affects and fantasies.
He also projected each representation into his perception of
me and felt his identification to be my experience.

MASOCHISTIC PROVOCATION: ACTING OUT

As a broad generalization one could say that in many ways
acting out represents a physical equivalent to the somatic symptoms. I shall simplify for the sake of exposition. As colitis patients give up their subjective representation of the parallel
physiological symptomatology, there is a coordinated loss of
physical symptoms. In virtually every patient I have seen successfully treated in psychoanalytic psychotherapy there is a shift
from smooth muscle, autonomic nervous system, and physiological activity to apparent voluntary activity—*acting out*—
smooth muscle to striated muscle, if you will. Usually there is
some back and forth shifting of activity in the process.

As patients achieve this level of ego integration, they have
a bit more insight into their own conflicts. They have learned

that they have control over their subjective representations of the gut, and, of course, effectively over the gut itself. Nevertheless, the same patients affectively remain to some extent in the infantile world of omnipotence and entitlement. Consequently one sees a familiar utilization of the subjective representations of acting out, facilitated by projections and projective identifications in the transference.

The affective manifestation of this subjective representation is a mild elation, a minimania accompanying the infantile fantasy of omnipotence, and the affective component of the illusion of entitlement gratification. As a matter of fact, Riviere (1936) and other Kleinians labeled it "manic" when they chose a name for the defense of omnipotent denial.

An interesting corollary is the observation that colitis patients often have a history of impulsive self-destructive activity before the onset of symptoms. (Though similar in nature, this preanalytic activity should not be called acting out. Acting out is defined by the therapeutic relationship. Outside the analytic context it is only, descriptively, impulsive and/or self-destructive action.) One of my patients had been a most self-destructive child and adolescent before the onset of his illness. He had an unbelievable number of injuries. To say he was accident-prone would be a monumental understatement.

This brings us to the recognition that when patients deny and avoid associations, they are responding to, and want to influence, the transference—or we might say influence their projected perceptions of, and identifications with, the psychoanalyst. The major problem here is the possibility that the analyst may unconsciously accept as valid the content of the projective identification—counteridentifying with the patient.

Once a patient has accepted a positive transference to the point of giving up symptoms (not a rebellious flight into health with symptomatic relief), there is little to worry about in the progress of the analysis. Now most of the analyst's anxieties about the damaging effects of acting out are countertransferential, representing a counteridentification with the patient's unconscious anxiety about impulses. It is of far greater importance to find the material to interpret this to the patient than it is to forbid, or even indicate any disapproval of, the activity. Not infrequently overt disapproval of a seemingly self-destructive activity produces a perverse reaction and induces the patient to rebelliously secretly repeat or intensify that activity (Hogan, 1983c).

Acting out represents attempts to deny the warnings of the superego and to indulge the derivatives of the forbidden impulse. The entire conflict is unconsciously projected onto the patient's perception of the psychoanalyst's state of mind and emotional responses. The inhibition, indulgence, provocation, disapproval, and potentiality of punishment are all present in the unconscious of the acting-out patient. One can see that the acting out may be one step elevated, but not too different in quality from, earlier provocations in the transference manipulations, which involved the exacerbations of symptoms.

As colitis patients give up their subjective representations of pathological colonic activity, they usually struggle with suicidal ideation, the content of which should be interpreted in context. My colleagues in psychosomatic practice and I have treated no colitis patient who indulged the impulse. None has attempted suicide with the exception of one who terminated psychoanalytic treatment in the initiatory stage, and who may have succeeded 18 months later. I have a very strong feeling that had we counteridentified and communicated anxiety to our patients, the results might have been quite different. A number of years ago a colleague who had had no experience with psychosomatic patients accepted one with ulcerative colitis for treatment. The patient attempted suicide and the analyst came to me for consultation. He had already hospitalized the patient and I could be of little help, but I recommended that he refer the patient to someone with experience in the treatment of ulcerative colitis. The patient took matters into her own hands and went to a psychiatrist of her own choice. Unfortunately, she did make another successful suicide attempt.

Most provocative acting out is of a less lethal nature. One patient developed ulcerative colitis with the perception of a specific deprivation in his marriage. He had acknowledged un-justified conscious but suppressed rage at his wife before relin-quishing his symptoms. He was able to give up the colitis after recognizing his preconscious sadistic destructive impulses to-ward this woman. However, before working it through and experiencing his ambivalence toward the maternal representa-tion, he indulged in his first and only extramarital affair. The acting out was a compromise gratification of his sadistic im-pulses. As one might predict, he unconsciously, but intention-ally, revealed his infidelity to his wife. The understandable con-sequences—accusations and temporary emotional abandon-ment—first precipitated profound shame and fear. As a recon-ciliation with his wife was slowly effected the patient's guilt broadened into a temporary but deep depression in which life did not seem to be worth living. He perceived himself as an ungrateful, worthless wretch.

The depression was relieved as he worked it out in the transference. It is here that we were able to understand the transference manipulations with their projective and identifi-catory mechanisms. He first blamed the analyst for not interfer-ing. When the patient accepted his own masochistic wishes for intervention, he then blamed the analysis for what he perceived to be his own irrational behavior. He was enraged at the frustra-tion supposedly imposed by the psychoanalyst. He felt that his acting-out behavior in response to the experienced frustration was entirely the responsibility of the psychoanalyst. We slowly worked out various aspects of his subjective battle with those fragmented precursors of his superego that he had projected upon me. In identifications maintained with those projected fragmented fantasies from the past he was both the passive recipient and the active perpetrator of my presumed judgments and fantasied forcible interventions. He unconsciously (and at times consciously) expected penetration, castration, abandon-ment. On the other side of his ambivalence he projected onto his perceptions of the analyst all the omnipotent loving protec-tive qualities of the maternal representation, with which he identified both passively and actively. It was repeatedly apparent that he maintained his original acting out with its complicated projective and identificatory content by splitting and denial. It would have been easy for me to interfere with cautionary advice at any time, but the entire transference content would have been lost. Following the affair, the discovery, the reconciliation, and his accusations was a relatively prolonged period of working out the content of, and associations to, the entire scenario. During this phase there were the same, but diminished, mental maneuvers of projection and identification.

Other provocative incidents of acting out by colitis patients are too numerous to document. They vary from complicated dramas such as the one above to repeated incidents of missed sessions or lateness, all justified and explained by projective and identificatory mechanisms. All involve pathological reanimations of infantile splitting in the context of contemporary environmental, or specific transference, pressures.

Significance of Countertransference

One might be justified in questioning my arbitrary division of countertransference phenomena into (1) denial and withdrawal, (2) symptom formation as a masochistic provocation, and (3) acting out as a masochistic provocation.

But in dealing with colitis, one can focus on two issues: (1) oft-observed denial with a suppression of fantasy and feeling, and (2) regular masochistic manipulation of the environmental projections whether by symptom or by action. All of the complex transference scenarios can be included under these generalities. One might even make a case for the denial and suppression of fantasy and feeling as an example of acting out (or to some, acting in). After all, there is activity involved in the inhibition of verbal production. In all events, such broad generalities (high orders of abstraction) have lost their explanatory value.

The transference allows the patient and the analyst to understand the patient's responses to the environment and to understand the primitive formative conflicts behind these responses. The significance of the countertransference is that the experience allows the psychoanalyst to understand the environment's responses to the patient and this is usually communicated back to the patient by inference or interpretation. When we attempt to treat a colitis patient, we find that in his or her unconscious both the subject and the environment are mutually provocative. The impulse provokes the fragmented superego and the punitive superego provokes the rebellious impulse. Both impulse and superego fragments are projected on the environment. One can expect that the psychoanalyst will be able to avoid the complex provocations and, in a suitable context, successfully communicate the information to the patient—assuming that the analyst possesses an adequate ration of feeling, experience, training, and intelligence.

Part IV
Afterword

Chapter 17
Afterword

Inflammatory bowel disease is a major public health problem and, if our epidemiological data continues on its present course, the medical profession will have to cope with larger and larger numbers of individuals suffering with ulcerative colitis and Crohn's disease. When a physician, or society, addresses a disease process there are a number of wishes and attempts: understand it, eradicate it, control it, immunize against it, and finally be able to forget it. When we can eradicate or inoculate against a pathogen, or where we can radically change variables such as the food supply, we contribute to the life expectancy in the underdeveloped nations of the world. Specific bacteria, viruses, or environmental factors do not seem to be the attackable enemies in many pathological conditions, including inflammatory processes in the gut.

To understand the complexities of most disease processes the medical scientist requires the input of specialists representing various sources of research data. Some investigators prefer to view the disease process and its treatment only from the province of their own field of observation, and to isolate understanding to the linguistic mode of their own data: "It is functional," "It is organic."

The unknowing professional or layperson has a right to be confused by the contradictions involved in the arbitrary presentations of "fact" that exclude the observations and successful therapeutic work of other groups of investigators. If the ideal treatment for every patient with the symptoms of an inflamed gut were psychoanalysis, it would not be available to all of these hypothetically treatable individuals. As with any disease, society does not contribute the talent, the money, or the time to universally dispense a conceivably ideal treatment. And, psychoanalytic psychotherapy, like any other approach, is not universally the ideal treatment.

Nevertheless, let us continue with our hypothesis. Let us assume that society were to furnish us with the wherewithal for such universal application of psychoanalytic psychotherapy. Society would find itself without the apparatus for the application. We do not have the supply of psychosomatically trained psychoanalysts to touch even a small segment of the epidemiological problem.

The lack of universal applicability or availability of treatment neither detracts from, nor proves the importance of any treatment modality. We cannot solve the public health problem and eradicate or repair inflammatory bowel disease in all patients or even a small proportion of them, but we can dispassionately examine relative merits and results of various therapeutic approaches.

Despite the time and effort necessary and the scarcity of psychosomatically trained psychiatrists, the psychoanalytic treatment of personality problems in appropriate patients remains an approach that can avoid mutilation and produce prolonged, often life-long physical remissions in a sizable number of individuals.

My chief purpose is to remind my medical colleagues that we can profitably treat many illnesses with more than simple technical mechanical manipulation of the human body and its chemistry. I have chosen, as a demonstration, a group of illnesses in which my co-investigators and I have a record of successful results with a psychoanalytic approach.

Above and beyond the frequency of therapeutic efficacy cited herein we have the most valuable and reliable source of data on the subjective conflicts in colitis patients available. Studies of physiology and behavior certainly contribute a lot to the parallel subjective world of observation. Testing and structured interviews can sometimes be informative. But only with the free spontaneous associations of a patient do we see drive and conflict in historical context and perspective. Let us once again remember that fragmentation, categorization, and labeling do not by themselves a science make. One should not worship our technical advances and forget the person.

We are still beginning to formulate and understand the laws of the psyche, but they are every bit as predictable and understandable as are the laws of physiology and biochemistry.

What about future research in the parallel areas of investigation, the 'subjective' and the 'physical'? Since so many contemporary studies erroneously insist on a temporal (causal) nature in the relationship inferred between these two separate areas of data retrieval, work needs to be done in this area.

In the subjective world, attempts to numerically quantify have been remarkably unproductive, and probably are inappropriate. In physical areas of observation, quantification and parcelization have been productive and appropriate in the structuring of concepts and data. Physiological and biochemical models and their accompanying technical efficiency have lent a rather seductive attraction to ideas of numerical weighting and quantification. Numerical quantification may well prove inadequate and inappropriate for the evaluation of the relative nature of subjective data.

For the present, one can be assured that in a reasonable percentage of appropriate patients, who remain in psychoanalytic psychotherapy until an agreed-upon termination of treatment, a properly trained psychoanalytic physician can expect gratifying results with a prolonged, perhaps life-long, remission.

References

Abraham, K. (1920), The narcissistic evaluation of excretory processes in dreams and neurosis. In: *Selected Papers on Psychoanalysis*, ed. E. Jones, tr. D. Bayan & A. Strachey. London: Hogarth Press & Institute of Psycho-Analysis, 1948, pp. 318–322.

——— (1921), Contribution to the theory of the anal character. In: *Selected Papers on Psychoanalysis*, ed. E. Jones, tr. D. Bayan & A. Strachey. London: Hogarth Press & Institute of Psycho-Analysis, 1948, pp. 370–392.

——— (1924), A short study of the development of the libido, viewed in the light of mental disorders: Part I, Manic-depressive states and the pregenital levels of the libido. In: *Selected Papers on Psychoanalysis*, ed. E. Jones, tr. D. Bayan & A. Strachey. London: Hogarth Press & Institute of Psycho-Analysis, 1948, pp. 418–503.

Adler, C. S., & Adler, S. M. (1989), A psychodynamic perspective on self-regulation in the treatment of psychosomatic disorders. In: *Psychosomatic Medicine: Theory, Physiology and Practice*, Vol. 2, ed. S. Cheren. Madison, CT: International Universities Press, pp. 841–898.

Aisenstein, M. (1993), Psychosomatic solution or somatic outcome: The man from Burma. Psychotherapy of a case of haemorrhagic rectocolitis. *Internat. J. Psycho-Anal.*, 74:371–381.

Alexander, F. (1939), Psychological aspects of medicine. *Psychosom. Med.*, 1:7–18.

——— (1950), *Psychosomatic Medicine. Its Principles and Application*. New York: Norton.

Allchin, W. H. (1885), A case of extensive ulceration of the colon. *Trans. Path. Soc. London*, 36:199–202.

Allison, M. C., & Pounder, R. E. (1984), Cyclosporin for Crohn's disease. *Lancet*, 1:902–903.

Almy, T. P. (1961a), Observations on the pathologic physiology of ulcerative colitis. *Gastroenterol.*, 41:299–306.

——— (1961b), Ulcerative colitis. *Gastroenterol.*, 41:391–400.

——— (1975), Psychiatric aspects of chronic ulcerative colitis and Crohn's colitis. In: *Inflammatory Bowel Disease*, ed. J. B. Kirsner & R. G. Shorter. Philadelphia: Lea & Febinger, pp. 37–46.

239

——— Hinkle, L. E., Jr., Berle, B., & Kern, F. (1949), Alterations in colonic functioning in man under stress: III. Experimental production of sigmoid spasm in patients with spastic constipation. *Gastroenterol.*, 12:437–449.

——— Kern, F., & Tulin, M. (1949), Alterations in colonic function in man under stress: II. Experimental production of sigmoid spasm in healthy persons. *Gastroenterol.*, 12:425–436.

——— Lewis, C. M. (1963), Ulcerative colitis. Report of progress based on recent literature. *Gastroenterol.*, 51:515–528.

——— Sherlock, P. (1966), Genetic aspects of ulcerative colitis and regional enteritis. *Gastroenterol.*, 51:757–761.

——— Tulin, M. (1947), Alterations in colonic functions in man under stress: I. Experimental production of changes simulating the "irritable colon." *Gastroenterol.*, 8:616–626.

Apfel, R. J., & Sifneos, P. E. (1979), Alexithymia: Concept and measurement. *Psychother. & Psychosom.*, 32:180–190.

Arlow, J. A., & Brenner, C. (1964), *Psychoanalytic Concepts and the Structural Theory*. New York: International Universities Press.

——— (1969), The psychopathology of the psychoses, a proposed revision. *Internat. J. Psycho-Anal.*, 50:5–14.

——— (1970), Discussion of "The psychopathology of the psychoses: A proposed revision." *Internat. J. Psycho-Anal.*, 51:159–166.

Atwell, J. D., Duthie, H. D., & Coligher, T. C. (1965), The outcome of Crohn's disease. *Brit. J. Surg.*, 52:966–972.

Babb, R. R. (1988a), Corticosteroids in ulcerative colitis: A skeptical view (editorial). *J. Clin. Gastroenterol.*, 10(4):365–367.

——— (1988b), The use of metronidazole (Flagyl) in Crohn's disease (editorial). *J. Clin. Gastroenterol.*, 10(5):479–481.

Banks, P. A., Present, D. H., & Steiner, P. (1983), *The Crohn's Disease and Ulcerative Colitis Fact Book*. New York: Charles Scribner & Sons for the National Foundation for Ileitis and Colitis.

Bayless, T. M. (1979), Environment vs. heredity in inflammatory bowel disease. In: *Inflammatory Bowel Disease: Experience and Controversy*, ed. B. I. Korelitz. Boston: John Wright PSG, 1982, pp. 21–24.

Bean, R. H. D. (1962), The treatment of chronic ulcerative colitis with 6-Mercaptopurine. *Med. J. Austral.*, 2:592–593.

——— (1966), Treatment of ulcerative colitis with anti-metabolites. *Brit. Med. J.*, 1:1081–1084.

Bernard, C. (1865), *Introduction a l'étude de la medicine experimentale*. Paris: J. B. Ballière.

——— (1878), Leçons sur les phenomenes de la vie communes aux animaux et aux vegetaux (Lectures on the phenomena of life common to animals and plants), tr. H. E. Hoff, R. Guillemin, & L. Guillemin. In: *American*

Lecture Series in the History of Medicine and Science. Paris: J. B. Ballière & Fils, 1878.

Binder, V. (1957), Trends in epidemiology of inflammatory bowel disease in Denmark/Scandinavia. In: *Inflammatory Bowel Diseases: Basic Research and Clinical Implications,* ed. H. Goebell, B. M. Peskar, & H. Malachow. Lancaster, U.K.: MTP Press, 1988, p. 237.

Bion, W. R. (1956), Development of schizophrenic thought. *Internat. J. Psycho-Anal.,* 37:344–346.

Bird, B. (1972), Notes on transference: Universal phenomenon and hardest part of analysis. *J. Amer. Psychoanal. Assn.,* 20:267–301.

Block, G. E., & Shraut, W. (1988), Complications of the surgical treatment of ulcerative colitis and Crohn's disease. In: *Inflammatory Bowel Disease,* 3rd ed., ed. J. B. Kirsner & R. G. Shorter. Philadelphia: Lea & Febinger, pp. 685–713.

Blum, H. P. (1977), The prototype of preoedipal reconstruction. *J. Amer. Psychoanal. Assn.,* 25:757–785.

Bowen, G. E., Irons, G. U., Jr., & Rhodes, J. B. (1966), Early experience with azathioprine in ulcerative colitis: A note of caution. *JAMA,* 195:460–464.

Boyer, L. B. (1961), Provisional evaluation of psycho-analysis with few parameters employed in the treatment of schizophrenia. *Internat. J. Psycho-Anal.,* 42:389–403.

——— (1979), Counter-transference with severely regressed patients. In: *Counter-transference: The Therapist's Contribution to the Therapeutic Situation,* ed. L. Epstein & A. H. Feiner. New York: Jason Aronson, pp. 347–374.

——— (1980), Working with the borderline patient. In: *Psychoanalytic Treatment of Schizophrenic, Borderline and Characterological Disorders,* ed. L. B. Boyer & P. L. Giovacchini. New York: Jason Aronson, pp. 173–208.

——— Giovacchini, P. L. (1980), *Psychoanalytic Treatment of Borderline and Characterological Disorders,* 2nd rev. ed. New York: Jason Aronson.

Bräutigam, W., & Rad, M. von, Eds. (1977), *Toward a Theory of Psychosomatic Disorders: Alexithymia, Pensée Opératoire, Psychosomatisches Phänomenon.* Proceedings of the 11th European Conference on Psychosomatic Research, Heidelberg 1976. Basel, Switzerland: S. Karger.

Brenner, C. (1976), *Psychoanalytic Technique and Psychic Conflict.* New York: International Universities Press.

——— (1979a), The components of psychic conflict and its consequences in mental life. *Psychoanal. Quart.,* 48:547–567.

——— (1979b), Working alliance, therapeutic alliance, and transference. *J. Amer. Psychoanal. Assn.,* 27(Suppl.):137–157.

——— (1982), *The Mind in Conflict.* New York: International Universities Press.

Breuer, J., & Freud, S. (1893–1895), Studies on hysteria. *Standard Edition,* 2. London: Hogarth Press, 1955.

Brooke, B. N., Hoffman, D. C., & Swarbuck, E. J. (1969), Azathioprine for Crohn's disease. *Lancet*, 2:612–614.

—— Javett, S. L., & Davison, O. W. (1970), Azathioprine for Crohn's disease. *Lancet*, 2:1050–1053.

Bruno, M. S. (1979), An internist's view of inflammatory bowel disease. In: *Inflammatory Bowel Disease: Experience and Controversy*, ed. B. I. Korelitz. Boston: John Wright PSG, 1982, pp. 5–8.

Bucaille, M. (1964), Selective frontal surgery in digestive pathology. *Le Scalpel J. Belge des Sci.*, 117:223–232.

Bynum, J. E., & Jacobson, E. D. (1988), Vascular diseases of the large bowel. In: *Diseases of the Colon, Rectum and Anal Canal*, ed. J. B. Kirsner & R. B. Shorter. Baltimore: Williams & Wilkins, pp. 537–546.

Cannon, W. B. (1929), *Bodily Changes in Pain, Hunger, Fear and Rage: An Account of Recent Researches into the Functions of Emotional Excitement*. New York: Appleton-Century-Crofts.

—— (1931), Studies on the conditions of activity in endocrine organs XXVII: Evidence that medulla adrenal secretion is not continuous. *Amer. J. Physiol.*, 98:447–453.

—— (1935), Stresses and strains of homeostasis. *Amer. J. Med. Sci.*, 189:1–14.

—— (1939), *The Wisdom of the Body*. New York: Norton.

Castelnuovo-Tedesco, P. (1966), Psychiatric observations on attacks of gout in a patient with ulcerative colitis. *Psychosom. Med.*, 28:781–788.

Cobb, S. (1963), Mind-body relationships. In: *The Psychological Basis of Medical Practice*, ed. H. I. Lief, V. F. Lief, & N. R. Lief. New York: Harper & Row, 1963, pp. 36–43.

Cook, M. O., & Dixon, M. F. (1973), An analysis of the reliability of detection and diagnostic value of various pathological features in Crohn's disease and ulcerative colitis. *Gut*, 14:255–262.

Crohn, B. B., Ginzburg, L., & Oppenheimer, C. D. (1932), Regional ileitis: A pathological and clinical entity. *JAMA*, 99:1323–1329.

—— Rosenberg, H. (1925), Sigmoidoscopic pictures of chronic ulcerative colitis (non-specific). *Amer. J. Med. Sci.*, 170:220–228.

Cushing, M. M. (1953), The psychoanalytic treatment of a man suffering with ulcerative colitis. *J. Amer. Psychoanal. Assn.*, 1:510–518.

Dalziel, T. K. (1913), Chronic interstitial enteritis. *Brit. Med. J.*, II:1068.

Daniels, G. E. (1935), Discussion of paper by Sullivan. *Amer. J. Dig. Dis. & Nutr.*, 2:656.

—— (1941), Practical aspects of psychiatric management in psychosomatic problems. *NY State J. Med.*, 41:1727–1732.

—— (1942), Psychiatric aspects of ulcerative colitis. *New Eng. J. Med.*, 226:178–184.

—— (1944), Non-specific ulcerative colitis as a psychosomatic disease. *Med. Clin. N. Amer.*, 28:593–602.

—— (1948), Psychiatric factors in ulcerative colitis. *Gastroenterol.*, 10:59–62.

—— O'Connor, J. F., Karush, A., Moses, L., Flood, C. A., & Lepore, M. (1962), Three decades in the observation and treatment of ulcerative colitis. *Psychosom. Med.*, 24:85–93.

Descartes, R. (1629), The world and treatise on man. In: *The Philosophical Writings of Descartes*, Vol. 1, tr. J. Cottingham, R. S. Stoothoff, & D. Murdoch. Cambridge: Cambridge University Press, 1990, pp. 79–108.

—— (1637), Discourse and essays. In: *The Philosophical Writings of Descartes*, Vol. 1, tr. J. Cottingham, R. S. Stoothoff, & D. Murdoch. Cambridge: Cambridge University Press, 1990, pp. 109–151.

—— (1641), Meditations on first philosophy. In: *The Philosophical Writings of Descartes*, Vol. 2, tr. J. Cottingham, R. S. Stoothoff, & D. Murdoch. Cambridge: Cambridge University Press, 1993, pp. 12–62.

—— (1644), Principles of philosophy. In: *The Philosophical Writings of Descartes*, Vol. 1, tr. J. Cottingham, R. S. Stoothoff, & D. Murdoch. Cambridge: Cambridge University Press, 1990, pp. 193–266.

—— (1649), The passions of the soul. In: *The Philosophical Writings of Descartes*, Vol I, trans. J. Cottingham, R. S. Stoothoff, & D. Murdock. Cambrige. Cambridge University Press, pp. 325–404.

Deutsch, F. (1922), On the formation of the conversion symptom. In: *On the Mysterious Leap from the Mind to the Body: A Study on the Theory of Conversion*, ed. F. Deutsch. New York: International Universities Press, 1959, pp. 59–72.

—— (1939), The production of somatic disease by emotional disturbance. In: *The Inter-relationship of Mind and Body*, ed. F. Kennedy, A. M. Frantz & C. C. Hare. Baltimore: Williams & Wilkins, pp. 271–292.

—— ed. (1953), *The Psychosomatic Concept in Psychoanalysis*. New York: International Universities Press.

—— Ed. (1959), *On the Mysterious Leap from the Mind to the Body: A Study on the Theory of Conversion*. New York: International Universities Press.

—— Semrad, E. V. (1959), Survey of Freud's writings on the conversion symptom. In: *On the Mysterious Leap from the Mind to the Body: A Study on the Theory of Conversion*, ed. F. Deutsch. New York: International Universities Press, pp. 27–46.

Deutsch, L. (1980), Psychosomatic medicine from a psychoanalytic viewpoint: A summary and review of four books. *J. Amer. Psychoanal. Assn.*, 28:653–702.

Dozois, R. R. & Kelly, K. A. (1988), Newer operations for ulcerative colitis and Crohn's disease. In: *Inflammatory Bowel Disease*, 3rd ed., ed. J. B. Kirsner & R. G. Shorter. Philadelphia: Lea & Febinger, pp. 655–683.

Dunbar, H. F. (1935), *Emotions and Bodily Changes: A Survey of the Literature of Psychosomatic Interrelationships (1910–1933)*. New York: Columbia University Press.

Eisenberg, R. L., Montgomery, C. K., & Margulis, A. R. (1979), Colitis in the elderly: Ischemic colitis mimicking ulcerative and granulomatous colitis. *Amer. J. Roentgenol.*, 133:1113–1118.

Eisenhammer, S. (1982), A case of acute fulminating ulcerative colitis: A complete cure and its urgent implications. *Amer. J. Proctol. Gastroenterol. & Colon & Rectal Surg.*, 33(6):10–11, 24.

Elliot, G. (1989), Stress and illness. In: *Psychosomatic Medicine: Theory, Physiology, and Practice*, Vol. 2, ed. S. Cheren. Madison, CT: International Universities Press, pp. 45–90.

Engel, G. L. (1952), Psychological aspects of the management of ulcerative colitis. *NY State J. Med.*, 22:2255–2261.

———— (1954a), Studies of ulcerative colitis: I. Clinical data bearing on the nature of the somatic process. *Psychosom. Med.*, 16:496–501.

———— (1954b), Studies of ulcerative colitis: II. The nature of the somatic processes and the adequacy of psychosomatic hypotheses. *Amer. J. Med.*, 16:416–433.

———— (1955), Studies of ulcerative colitis: III. The nature of the psychologic process. *Amer. J. Med.*, 19:231–256.

———— (1956), Studies of ulcerative colitis: IV. The significance of headaches. *Psychosom. Med.*, 18:334–346.

———— (1958), Studies of ulcerative colitis: V. Psychological aspects and their implications for treatment. *Amer. J. Dig. Dis.*, 33:315–337.

———— (1961a), Biological and psychologic features of the ulcerative colitis patient. *Gastroenterol.*, 40:313–322.

———— (1961b), Is grief a disease? A challenge for medical research. *Psychosom. Med.*, 23:18–22.

———— (1962), *Psychological Development in Health and Disease*. Philadelphia: Saunders.

———— (1967), The concept of psychosomatic disorder. *J. Psychosom. Res.*, 11:3–9.

———— (1973), Ulcerative colitis. In: *Emotional Factors in Gastrointestinal Illness*, ed. A. E. Lindner. New York: American Elsevier, pp. 99–112.

———— (1980), The clinical application of the biopsychosocial model. *Amer. J. Psychiat.*, 137(5):535–544.

———— Schmale, A. H., Jr. (1967), Psychoanalytic theory of somatic disorder: Conversion, specificity, and the disease onset situation. *J. Amer. Psychoanal. Assn.*, 15:345–365.

Fawaz, K. A., Glotzer, D. J., Goldman, H., Dickersin, G. R., Gross, W., & Patterson, J. F. (1976), Ulcerative colitis and Crohn's disease of the colon—A comparison of the long term postoperative courses. *Gastroenterol.*, 71:372–384.

———— ———— ———— ———— & Patterson, J. J. (1977), Ulcerative colitis and Crohn's disease of the colon: Their postoperative course. *Gastroenterology*, 72:775–779.

Feigl, H. (1950), The mind-body problem in the development of logical empiricism. In: *Readings in the Philosophy of Science*, ed. H. Feigl & M. Brodbeck. New York: Appleton-Century-Crofts, 1953, pp. 612–626.

―――― (1958), The "mental" and the "physical." In: *Concepts, Theories and the Mind-Body Problem*. Minnesota Studies in the Philosophy of Science. Minneapolis: University of Minnesota Press, pp. 370–497.

Fenichel, O. (1945a), Nature and classification of the so-called psychosomatic phenomena. In: *Collected Papers of Otto Fenichel*, 2nd series, ed. H. Fenichel & D. Rapaport. New York: Norton, 1954, pp. 305–323.

―――― (1945b), *The Psychoanalytic Theory of Neurosis*. New York: Norton.

Ferenczi, S. (1919), The phenomena of hysterical materialization: Thoughts on the conception of hysterical conversion and symbolism. In: *Further Contributions to the Theory and Technique of Psychoanalysis*, tr. J. I. Suttie et al. London: Hogarth Press, 1950, pp. 89–104.

Freud, S. (1891), *On Aphasia*. New York: International Universities Press, 1953.

―――― (1894), The neuro-psychoses of defence. *Standard Edition*, 3:45–61. London: Hogarth Press, 1962.

―――― (1895), Project for a scientific psychology. *Standard Edition*, 1:295–397. London: Hogarth Press, 1966.

―――― (1905), Fragment of an analysis of a case of hysteria. *Standard Edition*, 7:3–122. London: Hogarth Press, 1953.

―――― (1909), Notes upon a case of obsessional neurosis. *Standard Edition*, 10:153–249. London: Hogarth Press, 1955.

―――― (1913a), Totem and taboo. *Standard Edition*, 13:1–161. London: Hogarth Press, 1955.

―――― (1913b), On beginning the treatment (further recommendations on the technique of psycho-analysis I). *Standard Edition*, 12:121–144. London: Hogarth Press, 1958.

―――― (1914), On the history of the psycho-analytic movement. *Standard Edition*, 14:1–66. London: Hogarth Press, 1957.

―――― (1915), The unconscious. *Standard Edition*, 14:159–215. London: Hogarth Press, 1957.

―――― (1918 [1914]), From the history of an infantile neurosis. *Standard Edition*, 17:7–122. London: Hogarth Press, 1955.

―――― (1920), Beyond the pleasure principle. *Standard Edition*, 18:7–61. London: Hogarth Press, 1955.

―――― (1921), Group psychology and the analysis of the ego. *Standard Edition*, 18:69–143. London: Hogarth Press, 1955.

―――― (1923), The ego and the id. *Standard Edition*, 19:1–66. London: Hogarth Press, 1961.

―――― (1925), An autobiographical study. *Standard Edition*, 20:7–74. London: Hogarth Press, 1959.

———— (1933a), New introductory lectures on psycho-analysis and other works. *Standard Edition*, 22:7–182. London: Hogarth Press, 1964.

———— (1933b), Why war? (Einstein and Freud.) *Standard Edition*, 22:199–215. London: Hogarth Press, 1964.

———— (1937), Analysis terminable and interminable. *Standard Edition*, 23:216–253. London: Hogarth Press, 1964.

Freyberger, H. (1977), Supportive psychotherapeutic techniques in primary and secondary alexithymia. *Psychother. & Psychosom.*, 28:337–342.

Fullerton, D. T., Kollar, E. J., & Caldwell, A. B. (1962), A clinical study of ulcerative colitis. *JAMA*, 181:463–471.

Gilat, T. (1987), Epidemiology of IBD in central Israel 1970–1980. In: *Inflammatory Bowel Disease: Basic Research & Clinical Implications*, ed. H. Goebell, B. M. Peskar, & H. Malchow. Lancaster, U.K.: MTP Press, 1988, p. 239.

Gill, M. M. (1976), Metapsychology is not psychology. In: Psychology versus Metapsychology: Essays in Memory of George Klein. *Psychological Issues*, Vol. 9(4), Monograph 36, ed., M. M. Gill & P. S. Holzman. New York: International Universities Press, pp. 71–105.

———— Muslin, H. L. (1976), Early interpretation of transference. *J. Amer. Psychoanal. Assn.*, 24:779–793.

Giovacchini, P. L. (1975), Various aspects of the analytic process. In: *Tactics and Techniques in Psychoanalytic Therapy*, Vol. 2: *Counter-transference*, ed. P. L. Giovacchini, A. Flarscheim, & L. B. Boyer. New York: Jason Aronson, pp. 5–94.

———— (1977), The psychoanalytic treatment of the alienated patient. In: *New Perspectives on the Psychotherapy of the Borderline Adult*, ed. J. Masterson. New York: Brunner/Mazel, pp. 1–39.

———— (1979a), *Treatment of Primitive Mental States*. New York: Jason Aronson.

———— (1979b), Countertransference with primitive mental states. In: *Countertransference: The Therapist's Contribution to the Therapeutic Situation*, ed. L. Epstein & A. Feiner. New York: Jason Aronson, pp. 235–265.

Goldgraber, M. B., Humphreys, E. M., Kirsner, J. B., & Palmer, W. L. (1958), Carcinoma and ulcerative colitis: A clinical-pathological study, Parts I and II. *Gastroenterol.*, 34:809–846.

———— ———— ———— ———— (1959), Carcinoma and ulcerative colitis: A clinical-pathological study, Part III. *Gastroenterol.*, 36:613–630.

———— Kirsner, J. B. (1964), Carcinoma of the colon in ulcerative colitis. *Cancer*, 17:557–665.

Goodman, M. J., & Sparberg, M. (1978), *Ulcerative Colitis*. Clinical Gastroenterology Monograph Series, ed. J. M. Dietschy. New York: John Wiley.

Graham, D. T. (1967), Health, disease, and the mind-body problem: Linguistic parallelism. *Psychosom. Med.*, 29:52–71.

Greenacre, P. (1954), The role of transference: Practical considerations in relation to psychoanalytic therapy. *J. Amer. Psychoanal. Assn.*, 2:671–684.

Greenson, R. R. (1965), The working alliance and the transference neurosis. *Psychoanal. Quart.*, 34:155–181.

——— (1971), The "real" relationship between the patient and the psychoanalyst. In: *The Unconscious Today*, ed. M. Kanzer. New York: International Universities Press, pp. 213–232.

——— Wexler, M. (1969), The non-transference relationship in the psychoanalytic situation. *Internat. J. Psycho-Anal.*, 50:27–39.

Grinberg, L. (1979), Counter-transference and projective counter identifications. *Contemp. Psychoanal.*, 15:226–247.

Groddeck, G. W. (1912), Language. In: *The Meaning of Illness. Selected Psychoanalytic Writings of Georg Groddeck*, ed. L. Schacht, tr. G. Mander. New York: International Universities Press, 1977, pp. 248–264.

——— (1923), *The Book of the It: Psychoanalytic Letters to a Friend.* New York: Vintage, 1961.

Groen, J. (1947), Psychogenesis and psychotherapy of ulcerative colitis. *Psychosom. Med.*, 9:151–174.

——— (1951), Emotional factors in the etiology of internal disease. *Mt. Sinai J. Med.*, 18:71–79.

——— Bastiaans, J. (1954), Studies on ulcerative colitis: Personality structure, emotional conflict situations and effects of psychotherapy. In: *Modern Trends in Psychosomatic Medicine*, ed. D. O'Neill. New York: Hoeber, 1955, pp. 102–125.

——— Birnbaum, D. (1968), Conservative supportive treatment of severe ulcerative colitis. *Isr. J. Med. Sci.*, 4:130–139.

——— Van der Valk, J. M. (1956), Psychosomatic aspects of ulcerative colitis. *Practitioner*, 177:572–584.

Grotstein, J. S. (1981), *Splitting and Projective Identification.* New York: Jason Aronson.

——— (1983), Some perspectives on self psychology. In: *The Future of Psychoanalysis*, ed. A. Goldberg. New York: International Universities Press, pp. 165–201.

Gupta, S., Keshavazian, A., & Hodgson, H. J. F. (1984), Cyclosporin in ulcerative colitis. *Lancet*, 2:1277.

Hanauer, S. B., & Kirsner, J. B. (1989), Crohn's disease of the colon: Medical therapy. In: *Current Management of Inflammatory Bowel Disease*, ed. T. M. Bayless. Toronto: B. C. Decker, pp. 248–262.

Hawkins, C. (1983), Psychological problems and the management of patients with inflammatory bowel disease. In: *Inflammatory Bowel Disease*, ed. R. N. Allen, M. R. B. Keighley, J. Alexander-Williams & C. Hawkins. Edinburgh, Scotland/New York: Churchill Livingston, pp. 445–551.

Heath, R. G., Weber, J. J., Hogan, C. C., & Price, T. D. (1954), Metabolic change following destructive lesions in the forebrain of cats. In: *Studies in Schizophrenia: A Multidisciplinary Approach to Mind-Body Relationships*, ed R. G. Heath. Cambridge, MA: Harvard University Press, pp. 61–81.

Heimann, P. (1942), A contribution to the problem of sublimation and its relation to processes of internalization. *Internat. J. Psycho-Anal.*, 23:8–17.

Hofer, M. A. (1983), The mother-infant interaction as a regulator of infant physiology and behavior. In: *Symbiosis in Parent-Offspring Interactions*, ed. L. A. Rosenblum & H. Moltz. New York: Plenum, pp. 61–76.

———— (1984), Relationships as regulators: A psychobiologic perspective on bereavement. *Psychosom. Med.*, 46:183–197.

Hogan, C. C. (1952), Physiology of the caudate nucleus of the cat. New York: College of Physicians and Surgeons. Thesis for degree of Doctor of Medical Science, Columbia University College of Physicians and Surgeons, Health Sciences Library.

———— (1983a), Psychodynamics. In: *Fear of Being Fat: The Treatment of Anorexia Nervosa and Bulemia*, rev. ed., ed. C. P. Wilson, C. C. Hogan, & I. L. Mintz. New York: Jason Aronson, 1985, pp. 115–128.

———— (1983b), Object relations. In: *Fear of Being Fat: The Treatment of Anorexia Nervosa and Bulemia*, rev. ed., ed. C. P. Wilson, C. C. Hogan, & I. L. Mintz. New York: Jason Aronson, 1985, pp. 128–149.

———— (1983c), Transference. In: *Fear of Being Fat: The Treatment of Anorexia Nervosa and Bulemia*, rev. ed., ed. C. P. Wilson, C. C. Hogan, & I. L. Mintz. New York: Jason Aronson, 1985, pp. 158–168.

———— (1983d), Technical problems in psychoanalytic treatment. In: *Fear of Being Fat: The Treatment of Anorexia Nervosa and Bulemia*, rev. ed., ed. C. P. Wilson, C. C. Hogan, & I. L. Mintz. New York: Jason Aronson, 1985, pp. 197–215.

———— (1989), Inflammatory disease of the colon. In: *Psychosomatic Symptoms: Psychodynamic Treatment of the Underlying Personality Disorder*, ed. C. P. Wilson & I. L. Mintz. Northvale, NJ: Jason Aronson, pp. 367–399.

———— (1990), Possible technical modifications in the beginning phases of the psychoanalytic treatment of patients with psychosomatic symptoms. In: *On Beginning an Analysis*, ed. T. J. Jacobs & A. Rothstein. Madison, CT: International Universities Press, pp. 229–242.

———— (1992), Sexual identifications in anorexia nervosa. In: *Psychodynamic Technique in the Treatment of the Eating Disorders*, ed. C. P. Wilson, C. C. Hogan, & I. L. Mintz. Northvale, NJ: Jason Aronson, pp. 129–143.

Holt, R. R. (1967), Beyond vitalism and mechanism: Freud's concept of psychic energy. *Sci. & Psychoanal.*, 11:1–14.

Huizenga, K. A., & Schroeder, K. W. (1988), Gastrointestinal complications of ulcerative colitis. In: *Diseases of the Colon, Rectum, and Anal Canal*, ed. J. B. Kirsner & R. G. Shorter. Baltimore: Williams & Wilkins, pp. 257–280.

Jackson, D. D. (1946), The psychosomatic factors in ulcerative colitis. *Psychosom. Med.*, 8:278–280.

———— Yalom, I. (1966), Family research on the problems of ulcerative colitis. *Arch. Gen. Psychiat.*, 15:410–418.

Jewell, D. P. (1988), Systemic diseases and the large bowel. In: *Diseases of the Colon, Rectum, and Anal Canal*, ed. J. B. Kirsner & R. G. Shorter. Baltimore: Williams & Wilkins, pp. 549–560.

Karush, A., & Daniels, G. E. (1953). Ulcerative colitis: The psychoanalyses of two cases. *Psychosom. Med.*, 15:140–167.

―――――― O'Connor, J. F., & Stern, L. O. (1968), The response to psychotherapy in chronic ulcerative colitis: I. Pretreatment factors. *Psychosom. Med.*, 30:255–276.

―――― ―――― ―――― (1969), The response to psychotherapy in chronic ulcerative colitis: II. Factors arising from the therapeutic situation. *Psychosom. Med.*, 31:201–226.

―――― Daniels, G. E., Flood, C., & O'Connor, J. F. (1977), *Psychotherapy in Chronic Ulcerative Colitis*. Philadelphia: Saunders.

Kernberg, O. F. (1975), *Borderline Conditions and Pathological Narcissism*. New York: Jason Aronson.

―――― (1976), *Object-Relations Theory and Clinical Psychoanalysis*. New York: Jason Aronson.

Kidd, K. K., & Morton, L. A. (1989), The genetics of psychosomatic disorders. In: *Psychosomatic Medicine: Theory, Physiology, and Practice*, Vol. 1, ed. S. Cheren. Madison, CT: International Universities Press, pp. 385–424.

Kimball, C. P. (1981), *The Biopsychosocial Approach to the Patient*. Baltimore: Williams & Wilkins.

―――― (1989), On transitions: Psychosomatic medicine, liaison psychiatry and medicine and behavioral medicine. In: *Psychosomatic Medicine: Theory, Physiology, and Practice*, Vol. 2, ed. S. Cheren. Madison, CT: International Universities Press, pp. 765–812.

Kimura, A., & Sasagawa, S. (1984), Incidence of Crohn's disease in Japan. In: *Inflammatory Bowel Disease: Proceedings of the International Symposium on the Etiopathogenesis and Treatment of Inflammatory Bowel Disease*, ed. T. Shiraturi & H. Nakano. Tokyo: University of Tokyo Press, 1984, pp. 191–200.

Kirsner, J. B. (1980), Preface. In: *Recent Advances in Crohn's Disease: Proceedings of the Second International Workshop on Crohn's Disease*. Noordwijk, Leiden, June 25–28, 1980, ed. A. S. Pena, I. T. Watermum, C. C. Boothe, & W. Strober, p. xvii.

―――― Shorter, R. G. (1975), *Inflammatory Bowel Disease*. Philadelphia: Lea & Febinger.

―――― ―――― (1980), *Inflammatory Bowel Disease*, 2nd rev. ed. Philadelphia: Lea & Febinger.

―――― ―――― (1988), *Inflammatory Bowel Disease*, 3rd rev. ed. Philadelphia: Lea & Febinger.

Klein, H. S. (1965), Notes on a case of ulcerative colitis. *Internat. J. Psycho-Anal.*, 46:342–351.

Klein, M. (1955), On identification. In: *New Directions in Psychoanalysis*, ed. M. Klein, P. Heimann, & R. Money-Kryle. New York: Basic Books, pp. 309–345.

Knapp, P. H. (1981), Some contemporary contributions to the study of emotions. *J. Amer. Psychoanal. Assn.*, 35:205–248.

Koranyi, E. K. (1989), Physiology of stress reviewed. In: *Psychosomatic Medicine: Theory, Physiology and Practice*, Vol. 2, ed. S. Cheren. Madison, CT: International Universities Press, pp. 241–278.

Korelitz, B. I. (1977), Correspondence on: Ulcerative colitis and Crohn's disease of the colon: Their post operative course. *Gastroenterol.*, 72:775–779.

—— (1979), Evidence for Crohn's disease as an extensive process. In: *Inflammatory Bowel Disease: Experience & Controversy*, ed. B. I. Korelitz. Boston: John Wright PSG, 1982, pp. 9–14.

—— Gribetz, D. (1962), The prognosis of ulcerative colitis with onset in childhood: The steroid era. *Ann. Internal. Med.*, 57:592–597.

Korzybski, A. (1933), *Science and Sanity, An Introduction to Non-Aristotelian Systems and General Semantics*, 3rd ed. Lakeville, CT: International Non-Aristotelian Library, 1948.

Langman, J. S., & Logan, F. A. (1988), The epidemiology of human colonic diseases. In: *Diseases of the Colon, Rectum, and Anal Canal*, ed. J. B. Kirsner & R. G. Shorter. Baltimore: Williams & Wilkins, pp. 165–181.

Lauritsen, K., Laursen, L. S., Bukhave, K., & Rask-Madsen, J. (1987), Effect of therapy on erosanoid formation in inflammatory bowel disease. In: *Inflammatory Bowel Disease: Basic Research and Clinical Implications*, ed. H. Goebell, B. M. Peskar, & H. Malchow. Lancaster, U.K.: MTP Press, 1988, pp. 161–174.

Lefebvre, P. (1988), The psychoanalysis of a patient with ulcerative colitis: The impact of fantasy, affect, and the intensity of drives on the outcome of treatment. *Internat. J. Psycho-Anal.*, 69:43–53.

Lennard-Jones, J. (1981), Aetiology of non specific inflammatory bowel disease. In: *Colorectal Disease*, ed. J. Lennard-Jones, P. S. Thomas, R. J. Nicholls, & C. Williams. New York: Appleton-Century-Crofts, pp. 208–210.

Levitan, H. (1973), The etiological significance of deafness in ulcerative colitis. *Internat. J. Psychiat. Med.*, 4:379–387.

—— (1976), Psychological factors in the etiology of ulcerative colitis, objectlessness and rage. *Internat. J. Psychiat. Med.*, 7:221–226.

—— (1977), Infantile factors in two cases of ulcerative colitis. *Internat. J. Psychiat. Med.*, 8:185–190.

—— (1978), Implications from an unusual case of multiple psychosomatic illnesses. *Psychother. & Psychosom.*, 30:211–215.

—— (1981), Failure of defensive functions of the ego in dreams of psychosomatic patients. *Psychother. & Psychosom.*, 36:1–7.

———— (1982), Explicit incestuous motifs in psychosomatic patients. *Psychother. & Psychosom.*, 37:22–25.

———— (1989a), Onset situation in three psychosomatic illnesses. In: *Psychosomatic Medicine: Theory, Physiology and Practice*, Vol. 1, ed. S. Cheren. Madison, CT: International Universities Press, pp. 119–134.

———— (1989b), Failure of the defensive functions of the ego in psychosomatic patients. In: *Psychosomatic Medicine: Theory, Physiology and Practice*, Vol. 1, ed. S. Cheren. Madison, CT: International Universities Press, pp. 135–157.

Lewin, B. D. (1950), *The Psychoanalysis of Elation.* New York: Norton.

Lightdale, C. J., & Sherlock, P. (1988), Neoplasia and gastrointestinal malignancy in inflammatory bowel disease. In: *Diseases of the Colon, Rectum, and Anal Canal*, ed. J. B. Kirsner & R. G. Shorter. Baltimore: Williams & Wilkins, pp. 281–298.

Lindemann, E. (1945), Psychiatric problems in the conservative treatment of ulcerative colitis. *Arch. Neurol. & Psychiat.*, 53:322–324.

———— (1950), Modifications in the course of ulcerative colitis in relationship to changes in life situations and reaction patterns. *Proc. Assn. Res. Nerv. Ment. Dis.*, 29:706–723.

Lipowski, Z. J., Lipsitt, D. R., & Whybrow, P. C., Eds. (1977), *Psychosomatic Medicine: Current Trends and Clinical Applications.* New York: Oxford University Press.

Lockhart-Mummery, H. E., & Morson, B. C. (1960), Crohn's disease (regional enteritis) of the large intestine and its distinction from ulcerative colitis. *Gut*, 1:87–105.

Loewenstein, R. M. (1969), Developments in the theory of transference in the last fifty years. *Internat. J. Psycho-Anal.*, 50:583–588.

Lolas, F., & Rad, M. von (1989), Alexithymia. In: *Psychosomatic Medicine: Theory, Physiology and Practice*, Vol. 1, ed. S. Cheren. Madison, CT: International Universities Press, pp. 189–237.

Mahler, M. S. (1967), On human symbiosis and the vicissitudes of individuation. In: *The Selected Papers of Margaret S. Mahler*, Vol. 2: *Separation-Individuation.* New York: Jason Aronson, 1979, pp. 77–97.

Măratka, Z. (1986), Pathogenesis and etiology of inflammatory bowel disease. In: *Inflammatory Bowel Disease: Some International Data and Reflections*, ed. F. T. deDombel, J. Myren, A. D. Boucher, & G. Watkinson. New York: Oxford University Press, pp. 29–65.

Marty, P. (1976), *L'ordre psychosomatique les souvements individuels de vie et de mort.* Paris: Payot.

———— DeBray, R. (1989), The current concepts of character disturbance. In: *Psychosomatic Medicine: Theory, Physiology and Practice*, Vol. 1, ed. S. Cheren. Madison, CT: International Universities Press, pp. 159–188.

———— de M'Uzan, M. (1963), La Pensée opératoire. *Rev. Franc. Psychoanal.*, 27:345–356.

—— —— David, C. (1963), *L'Investigation psychosomatique*. Paris: Presses Universitaires de France.

Mason, J. W. (1971), A re-evaluation of the concept of "non-specificity" in stress theory. *J. Psychiat. Res.*, 8:323–333.

McDougall, J. (1982a), Alexithymia: A psychoanalytic viewpoint. *Psychother. & Psychosom.*, 38:81–90.

—— (1982b), Alexithymia, psychosomatosis, and psychosis. *Internat. J. Psychoanal. Psychother.*, 9:379–388.

—— (1985), *Theatres of the Mind: Illusion and Truth on the Psychoanalytic Stage*. New York: Basic Books.

—— (1989), *Theatres of the Body: A Psychoanalytic Approach to Psychosomatic Illness*. New York: Norton.

McKegney, P. P., Gordon, R. O., & Levine, S. M. (1970), A psychosomatic comparison of patients with ulcerative colitis and Crohn's disease. *Psychosom. Med.*, 32:153–166.

Mendelhoff, A. T., & Calkins, B. M. (1988), Epidemiology in inflammatory bowel disease. In: *Inflammatory Bowel Disease*, 3rd ed., ed. J. B. Kirsner & R. G. Shorter. Philadelphia: Lea & Febinger, pp. 3–34.

Mintz, I. L. (1989), Treatment of a case of anorexia and severe asthma. In: *Psychosomatic Symptoms: Psychodynamic Treatment of the Underlying Personality Disorder*, ed. C. P. Wilson & I. L. Mintz. Northvale, NJ: Jason Aronson, pp. 251–307.

Mirsky, I. A. (1953), Psychoanalysis and the biological sciences. In: *Twenty Years in Psychoanalysis*, ed. F. Alexander & H. Ross. New York: Norton, pp. 155–181.

—— (1957), The psychosomatic approach to the etiology of clinical disorders. *Psychosom. Med.*, 19:424.

Morgagni, G. (1769), *De Sedibus et Causis Morborum per Anatomen Indagatis Libri Quinque*. New York: Hafner, 1960.

Murray, C. D. (1930a), Psychogenic factors in the etiology of colitis and bloody diarrhea. *Amer. J. Med. Sci.*, 180:239–248.

—— (1930b), A brief psychological analysis of a patient with ulcerative colitis. *J. Nerv. & Ment. Dis.*, 72:617–627.

Murray, J. M. (1964), Narcissism and the ego ideal. *J. Amer. Psychoanal. Assn.*, 12:477–511.

Mushatt, C. (1954), Psychological aspects of non-specific ulcerative colitis. In: *Recent Developments in Psychosomatic Medicine*, ed. E. R. Wittkower & B. A. Cleghorn. Philadelphia: Lippincott, pp. 345–363.

—— (1959), Loss of sensory perception determining the choice of symptom. In: *On the Mysterious Leap from the Mind to the Body: A Study on the Theory of Conversion*, ed. F. Deutsch. New York: International Universities Press, 1959, pp. 201–234.

—— (1975), Mind-body-environment: Toward understanding the impact of loss on psyche and soma. *Psychoanal. Quart.*, 44:81–106.

—— (1989), Loss, separation and psychosomatic illness. In: *Psychosomatic Symptoms: Psychodynamic Treatment of the Underlying Personality Disorder*, ed. C. P. Wilson & I. L. Mintz. Northvale, NJ: Jason Aronson, pp. 33–61.

Nemiah, J. C., Freyberger, S., & Sifneos, P. E. (1976), Alexithymia: A view of the psychosomatic process. In: *Modern Trends in Psychosomatic Medicine*, Vol. 3, ed. O. Hill. London: Butterworth, pp. 430–439.

—— Sifneos, P. E. (1970), Affect and fantasy in patients with psychosomatic disorders. In: *Modern Trends in Psychosomatic Medicine*, Vol. 2, ed. O. W. Hill. New York: Appleton-Century-Crofts, pp. 26–34.

Niederland, W. G. (1956), Clinical observation on the "Little Man" phenomenon. *The Psychoanalytic Study of the Child*, 11:381–395. New York: International Universities Press.

—— (1965), Narcissistic ego impairment in patients with early physical malformations. *The Psychoanalytic Study of the Child*, 20:518–534. New York: International Universities Press.

Norris, H. T. (1977), Ischemic bowel disease: Its spectrum. In: *The Gastrointestinal Tract*, ed. J. H. Hardley, B. C. Morson, & M. R. Abell. Baltimore: Williams & Wilkins, pp. 15–30.

North, C. S., Clouse, R. E., Spitznagel, E. L., & Alpers, D. H. (1990), The relation of ulcerative colitis to psychiatric factors: A review of findings and methods. *Amer. J. Psychiat.*, 147:973–981.

Patterson, D. J., Ball, T. J., & Witske, K. E. (1988), Methotrexate inducing clinical and histological remission in retractory inflammatory bowel disease (abstract). *Gastroenterol.*, 94(Part 2):9238.

Petras, R. E., Bona, S. J., McGonagle, B., & Fazio, V. W. (1987), "Pouchitis" in patients with continent ileostomy: A histological study. In: *Inflammatory Bowel Disease: Current Status and Future Approach*, ed. R. MacDermott. Amsterdam, Netherlands: Excerpta Medica, 1988, pp. 699–704.

Porder, M. (1987), Projective identification: An alternative hypothesis. *Psychoanal. Quart.*, 56:431–451.

Present, D. H. (1989), 6-Mercaptopurine and other immunosuppressive agents in the treatment of Crohn's disease and ulcerative colitis. *Gastroenterol. Clin. N. Amer.*, 18(1):57–71.

—— Korelitz, B. I., Wisch, N., Glass, J. L., Sacher, D. B., & Pasternack, B. S. (1980), Treatment of Crohn's disease with 6-Mercaptopurine. A long-term, random, double-blind study. *New Eng. J. Med.*, 302:981–987.

—— Meltzer, S. J., Krumholz, M. P., Wolke, A., & Korelitz, B. I. (1989), 6-Mercaptopurine in the management of inflammatory bowel disease: Short and long term toxicity. *Annals Internal Med.*, 111(8):641–649.

Price, L. (1954), *Dialogues of Alfred North Whitehead as Recorded by Lucien Price*. Boston: Little, Brown.

Prugh, D. G. (1950), Variations in attitudes, behavior and feeling states as exhibited in the play of children during modifications in the course of ulcerative colitis. *Res. Nerv. Ment. Dis.*, 29:692–705.

254 REFERENCES

——— (1951), The influence of emotional factors on the clinical course of ulcerative colitis in children. *Gastroenterol.*, 18:339–354.

Purrmann, J. (1987), Genetic aspects of inflammatory bowel disease. In: *Inflammatory Bowel Disease: Basic Research & Clinical Implications*, ed. H. Goebell, B. M. Peskar, & H. Malchow. Norwell, MA: MTP Press, 1988, pp. 203–213.

Quinn, T. C., & Schuffler, M. D. (1988), The clinical aspects of specific infections of the large bowel and anal canal, including the "gay bowel syndrome." In: *Diseases of the Colon, Rectum and Anal Canal*, ed. J. B. Kirsner & R. G. Shorter. Baltimore: Williams & Wilkins, pp. 439–481.

Raab, B., Fretzin, D., Bronson, D., Scott, M., Roenak, H., & Medenica, M. (1983), Epidermolysis bullosa acquisita and inflammatory bowel disease. *JAMA*, 250:1746–1748.

Reiser, M. F. (1975), Changing theoretical concepts in psychosomatic medicine. In: *American Handbook of Psychiatry*, Vol. 4, ed. M. Reiser. New York: Basic Books, pp. 477–497.

——— (1978), Psychoanalysis in patients with psychosomatic disorders. In: *Psychotherapeutics in Medicine*, ed. T. B. Karasu & R. I. Steinmuller. New York: Grune & Stratton, pp. 63–74.

Riviere, J. (1936), A contribution to the analysis of negative therapeutic reaction. *Internat. J. Psycho-Anal.*, 17:304–320.

Rosenfeld, H. A. (1952), Notes on the psycho-analysis of the super-ego conflict of an acute schizophrenic patient. *Internat. J. Psycho-Anal.*, 33:111–131.

Roth, J. L. A. (1976), Ulcerative colitis. In: *Gastroenterology*, Vol. 2, 3rd ed., ed. E. L. Bockus, J. E. Berk, W. S. Haubrich, M. Kalser, J. L. A. Roth, & F. Vilardell. Philadelphia: Saunders, pp. 645–749.

Ruderman, W. B. (1987), Pouchitis: A novel form of idiopathic ileitis. In: *Inflammatory Bowel Disease: Current Status and Future Approach*, ed. R. MacDermott. Amsterdam, Netherlands: Excerpta Medica, 1988, pp. 695–698.

Russell, B. (1929), On the notion of cause with application to the free will problem. In: *Readings in the Philosophy of Science*, ed. H. Feigl & M. Brodbeck. New York: Norton, pp. 387–418.

Sacher, D. B., Greenstein, A. J., & Janowitz, H. D. (1977), Correspondence. *Gastroenterol.*, 72:777.

Sandler, J., Dare, C., & Holder, A. (1973), *The Patient and the Analyst*. New York: International Universities Press.

Sarnoff, C. (1989), Early psychic stress and psychosomatic disease. In: *Psychosomatic Symptoms: Psychodynamic Treatment of the Underlying Personality Disorder*, ed. C. P. Wilson & I. L. Mintz. Northvale, NJ: Jason Aronson, pp. 83–103.

Savitt, R. A. (1963), Psychosomatic studies on addiction: Ego structure in narcotic addiction. *Psychoanal. Quart.*, 32:43–57.

——— (1969), Transference, somatization, and symbiotic needs. *J. Amer. Psychoanal. Assn.*, 17:1030–1054.

——— (1977), Conflict and somatization: Psychoanalytic treatment of the psychophysiologic response in the digestive tract. *Psychoanal. Quart.*, 46:605–622.

Schur, M. (1955), Comments on the metapsychology of somatization. *The Psychoanalytic Study of the Child*, 10:110–164. New York: International Universities Press.

Schwaber, E. A. (1990), Interpretation and therapeutic action of psychoanalysis. *Internat. J. Psycho-Anal.*, 71:229–240.

Schwartz, G. E. (1977), Psychosomatic disorders and biofeedback: A psychobiological model of disregulation. In: *Psychopathology: Experimental Models*, ed. J. D. Maser & M. E. P. Seligman. San Francisco: W. H. Freeman, pp. 220–307.

——— (1979), Disregulation and systems theory: A biobehavioral framework for biofeedback and behavioral medicine. In: *Biofeedback and Self-Regulation*, ed. N. Birbaumer & H. D. Kimmel. Hillsdale, NJ: Lawrence Erlbaum, pp. 19–48.

——— (1981), A systems analysis of psychobiology and behavior therapy: Implications for behavioral medicine. *Psychother. & Psychosom.*, 36:159–184.

——— (1983), Disregulation theory and disease: Applications to the repression/cerebral disconnection/cardiovascular disorder hypothesis. *Internat. Rev. Appl. Psychol.*, 32:95–118.

——— (1989), Disregulation theory and disease: Toward a general model for psychosomatic medicine. In: *Psychosomatic Medicine: Theory, Physiology and Practice*, Vol. 1, ed. S. Cheren. Madison, CT: International Universities Press, pp. 91–117.

Schwartz, J. T., & Graham, D. Y. (1988), Diverticular disease of the large intestine. In: *Diseases of the Colon, Rectum, and Anal Canal*, ed. J. B. Kirsner & R. G. Shorter. Baltimore: Williams & Wilkins, 1988, pp. 519–536.

Searle, J. (1984), *Minds, Brains and Science*. Cambridge, MA: Harvard University Press.

Searles, H. F. (1963), Transference psychosis in the psychotherapy of chronic schizophrenia. In: *Collected Papers on Schizophrenia and Related Subjects*. New York: International Universities Press, 1969, pp. 654–716.

——— (1966), Feelings of guilt in the psychoanalyst. *Psychiat.*, 29:319–323.

——— (1975), The patient as therapist to his analyst. In: *Tactics and Techniques in Psychoanalytic Therapy*, Vol. 2, ed. P. L. Giovacchini. New York: Jason Aronson, pp. 95–151.

——— (1979), The analyst's experience with jealousy. In: *Countertransference: The Therapist's Contribution to the Therapeutic Situation*, ed. L. E. Epstein & A. H. Feiner. New York: Jason Aronson, pp. 305–327.

Selye, H. (1936), A syndrome produced by diverse nocuous agents. *Nature*, 138:32.

—— (1950), *The Physiology and Pathology of Exposure to Stress*. Montreal: Actea.

—— (1956), *The Stress of Life*. New York: McGraw-Hill.

—— (1974), *Stress Without Distress*. Toronto: McLelland & Stewart.

Shivananda, S., Hordijk, M. L., Peña, A. S., Ruitenberg, E. J., & Mayberry, J. F. (1987), Epidemiology of inflammatory bowel disease in regio Leiden, The Netherlands. In: *Inflammatory Bowel Diseases: Basic Research and Clinical Implications*, ed. H. Goebell, B. M. Peskar, & H. Malchow. Lancaster, U.K.: MTP Press, 1988, pp. 245–247.

Sidaron, J. (1986), The protean complications of inflammatory bowel disease. In: *Inflammatory Bowel Disease: Some International Data and Reflections*, ed. F. deDombel, J. Myren, I. Boucher, & G. Watkinson. New York: Oxford University Press, pp. 161–246.

Sifneos, P. E. (1972), *Short-Term Psychotherapy and Emotional Crisis*. Cambridge, MA: Harvard University Press.

—— (1973), The prevalence of "alexithymic" characteristics in psychosomatic patients. *Psychother. & Psychosom.*, 22:255–262.

Sperling, M. (1946), Psychoanalytic study of ulcerative colitis in children. *Psychoanal. Quart.*, 15:302–329.

—— (1949a), The role of the mother in psychosomatic disorders in children. *Psychosom. Med.*, 11:377–385.

—— (1949b), Problems in the analysis of children with psychosomatic disorders. *J. Child. Behav.*, 1:12–17.

—— (1952), Psychotherapeutic techniques in psychosomatic medicine. In: *Specialized Techniques in Psychotherapy*, ed. G. Bychowski & J. L. Demoert. New York: Basic Books, pp. 279–301.

—— (1955a), Observations from the treatment of children suffering from nonbloody diarrhea or mucous colitis. *J. Hillside Hosp.*, 4:25–31.

—— (1955b), Psychosis and psychosomatic illness. *Internat. J. Psycho-Anal.*, 36:320–327.

—— (1957), The psychoanalytic treatment of ulcerative colitis. *Internat. J. Psycho-Anal.*, 38:341–349.

—— (1960), Unconscious phantasy of life and object relations in ulcerative colitis. Symposium on disturbances of the digestive tract. *Internat. J. Psycho-Anal.*, 41:450–455.

—— (1961), Psychosomatic disorders. In: *Adolescents: Psychoanalytic Approach to Problems and Therapy*, ed. S. Lorand & H. I. Schneer. New York: Hoeber, pp. 202–216.

—— (1963), Psychoanalytic study of bronchial asthma in children. In: *The Asthmatic Child: Psychosomatic Approach to Problems and Treatment*, ed. H. Schneer. New York: Harper & Row, pp. 138–165.

———— (1964), A case of ophidophilia: A clinical contribution to snake symbolism and a supplement to the psychoanalytic study of ulcerative colitis in children. *Internat. J. Psycho-Anal.*, 45:227–233.

———— (1967), Transference neurosis in patients with psychosomatic disorders. *Psychoanal. Quart.*, 36:342–355.

———— (1968), Acting-out behavior and psychosomatic symptoms: Clinical and theoretical aspects. *Internat. J. Psycho-Anal.*, 49:250–253.

———— (1969), Ulcerative colitis in children: Current views and therapies. *J. Amer. Acad. Child Psychiat.*, 8:336–352.

———— (1973), Conversion hysteria and conversion symptoms: Revision of classification and concepts. *J. Amer. Psychoanal. Assn.*, 21:745–771.

———— (1978a), Psychosomatic study of ulcerative colitis. In: *Psychosomatic Disorders in Childhood*, ed. O. E. Sperling. New York: Jason Aronson, pp. 77–98.

———— (1978b), Ulcerative colitis in children: Current views and therapies. In: *Psychosomatic Disorders in Childhood*, ed. O. E. Sperling. New York: Jason Aronson, pp. 6–119.

Sperling, O. E. (1978a), The concept of psychosomatic disease. In: *Psychosomatic Disorders in Childhood*, ed. O. E. Sperling. New York: Jason Aronson, pp. 3–10.

———— (1978b), A case of angioneurotic edema. In: *Psychosomatic Disorders in Childhood*, ed. O. E. Sperling. New York: Jason Aronson, pp. 353–357.

Sterba, R. F. (1934), The fate of the ego in analytic therapy. *Internat. J. Psycho-Anal.*, 15:117–126.

Stone, L. (1967), The psychoanalytic situation and transference: Postscript to an earlier communication. *J. Amer. Psychoanal. Assn.*, 15:3–58.

Stout, C., & Snyder, R. L. (1969), Ulcerative colitis like lesion in Siamang gibbons. *Gastroenterol.*, 57:256–261.

Sullivan, A. J. (1935), Psychogenic factors in ulcerative colitis. *Amer. J. Dig. Dis. & Nutr.*, 2:651–656.

———— Chandler, A. C. (1932), Ulcerative colitis of psychogenic origin: A report of 6 cases. *Yale J. Biol. Med.*, 4:779–796.

Summers, K. W., Switz, D. M., & Sessions, J. T. (1979), National comparative Crohn's diseases study: Results of drug treatment. *Gastroenterol.*, 77:847–869.

Taylor, G. J. (1987), *Psychosomatic Medicine and Contemporary Psychoanalysis.* Madison, CT: International Universities Press.

Thayer, W. R., & DeNucci, T. (1988), Miscellaneous diseases of the large bowel and anal canal. In: *Diseases of the Colon, Rectum and Anal Canal*, ed. J. B. Kirsner & R. G. Shorter. Baltimore: Williams & Wilkins, pp. 561–594.

Usdin, E., Hamburg, D. A., & Barchas, J. D., eds. (1977), *Neuroregulators and Psychiatric Disorders: Proceedings Conference on Neuroregulators, and Hypothesis of Psychiatric Disorders (1976).* New York: Oxford University Press.

Utsunomiya, T., Shinohara, H., Kitahora, T., Suzuki, K., & Yokota, A. (1982), Epidemiological study on the incidence of idiopathic proctocolitis in Japan: An enquête study. In: *Inflammatory Bowel Disease: Proceedings of the International Symposium on Etiopathogenesis and Treatment of Inflammatory Bowel Disease*, ed. T. Shiraturi & H. Nakano. Tokyo: University of Tokyo Press, 1984, pp. 185–189.

Volkan, V. D. (1965), The observation of the "little man" phenomenon in a case of anorexia nervosa. *Brit. J. Med. Psychol.*, 38:299–311.

——— (1975), *Primitive Internalized Object Relations: A Clinical Study of Schizophrenic, Borderline and Narcissistic Patients*. New York: International Universities Press.

von Bertalanffy, L. (1964), The mind-body problem: A new view. *Psychosom. Med.*, 26:29–45.

——— (1968), *General Systems Theory*. New York: Braziller.

Weiner, H. (1970), The mind-body unity in the light of recent physiological evidence. *Psychother. & Psychosom.*, 18:117–122.

——— (1972), Some comments on the transduction of experience by the brain: Implications for our understanding of the relationship of mind to body. *Psychosom. Med.*, 34:355–380.

——— (1977), *Psychobiology and Human Disease*. New York: Elsevier.

——— (1982), The prospects for psychosomatic medicine. Selected topics. *Psychosom. Med.*, 44:491–517.

——— Fawzy, I. (1989), An interactive model of health, disease and illness. In: *Psychosomatic Medicine: Theory, Physiology and Practice*, Vol. 1, ed. S. Cheren. Madison, CT: International Universities Press, pp. 9–44.

Weinstock, H. I. (1962), Successful treatment of ulcerative colitis by psychoanalysis. A survey of 28 cases with follow-up. *J. Psychosom. Res.*, 6:243–249.

——— (1966), Hospital psychotherapy in severe ulcerative colitis: The ineffectiveness in preventing surgical measures and recurrences. *Arch. Gen. Psychiat.*, 4:509–512.

White, W. H. (1888), On simple ulcerative colitis and other rare intestinal ulcers. *Guys Hosp. Rep.*, 30:131–162.

Whitehead, A. N. (1938), Modes of thought. In: *Alfred North Whitehead: An Anthology*, ed. F. S. C. Northrop & M. W. Gross. New York: Macmillan, 1953, pp. 861–924.

Whorf, B. L. (1941a), Language, mind, and reality. In: *Language, Thought, and Reality: Selected Writings of Benjamin Lee Whorf*, ed. J. B. Carroll. Cambridge, MA: The Technology Press of Massachusetts Institute of Technology and (New York) John Wiley, 1956, pp. 246–270.

——— (1941b), Languages and logic. In: *Language, Thought, and Reality: Selected Writings of Benjamin Lee Whorf*, ed. J. B. Carroll. Cambridge, MA: The Technology Press of Massachusetts Institute of Technology and (New York) John Wiley, 1956, pp. 233–245.

Wilks, S. (1859a), *Lectures on Pathological Anatomy*. London: Churchill.
——— (1859b), Morbid appearance in the intestines of Miss Bankes. *Med. Times & Gazette*, pp. 264–265.
——— Moxon, W. (1875), *Lectures on Pathological Anatomy*. London: Churchill.
Wilson, C. P. (1983a), Contrasts in the analysis of bulimic and abstaining anorexics. In: *Fear of Being Fat: The Treatment of Anorexia Nervosa and Bulemia*, rev. ed., ed. C. P. Wilson, C. C. Hogan, & I. L. Mintz. New York: Jason Aronson, 1985, pp. 169–193.
——— (1983b), Dream interpretation. In: *Fear of Being Fat: The Treatment of Anorexia Nervosa and Bulemia*, rev. ed., ed. C. P. Wilson, C. C. Hogan, & I. L. Mintz. New York: Jason Aronson, 1985, pp. 245–254.
——— (1989a), Dream interpretation. In: *Psychosomatic Symptoms: Psychodynamic Treatment of the Underlying Personality Disorder*, ed. C. P. Wilson & I. L. Mintz. Northvale, NJ: Jason Aronson, pp. 133–145.
——— (1989b), Ego functioning in psychosomatic disorder. In: *Psychosomatic Symptoms: Psychodynamic Treatment of the Underlying Personality Disorder*, ed. C. P. Wilson & I. L. Mintz. Northvale, NJ: Jason Aronson, pp. 13–32.
——— (1989c), Family psychopathology. In: *Psychosomatic Symptoms: Psychodynamic Treatment of the Underlying Personality Disorder*, ed. C. P. Wilson & I. L. Mintz. Northvale, NJ: Jason Aronson, pp. 63–82.
——— (1989d), Projective identification. In: *Psychosomatic Symptoms: Psychodynamic Treatment of the Underlying Personality Disorder*, ed. C. P. Wilson & I. L. Mintz. Northvale, NJ: Jason Aronson, pp. 105–132.
——— (1989e), Parental overstimulation in asthma. In: *Psychosomatic Symptoms: Psychodynamic Treatment of the Underlying Personality Disorder*, ed. C. P. Wilson & I. L. Mintz. Northvale, NJ: Jaron Aronson, pp. 327–349.
——— Hogan, C. C., & Mintz, I. L., Eds. (1983), *Fear of Being Fat: The Treatment of Anorexia Nervosa and Bulemia*, rev. ed. New York: Jason Aronson, 1985.
——— ——— ——— Eds. (1992), *Psychodynamic Technique in the Treatment of Eating Disorders*. Northvale, NJ: Jason Aronson.
——— Mintz, I. L., Eds. (1989), *Psychosomatic Symptoms: Psychodynamic Treatment of the Underlying Personality Disorder*. Northvale, NJ: Jason Aronson.
Winkelman, E. I., & Brown, C. H. (1965), Nitrogen mustard in the treatment of chronic ulcerative colitis and regional enteritis: A preliminary report. *Cleveland Clinic. Quart.*, 32:165–174.
Winnicott, D. W. (1965), *The Maturational Processes and the Facilitating Environment*. New York: International Universities Press.
Wittkower, E. D., & Warnes, H., eds. (1977), *Psychosomatic Medicine: The Clinical Applications*. Haggerstown, MO: Harper & Row.
Wolff, H. G. (1950), Life stress and bodily disease: A formulation. In: *Life Stress and Bodily Disease: Proceedings of the Association for Research in Nervous and Mental Disease*, ed. H. Wolff, S. Wolff, & C. E. Hare. Baltimore: Williams & Wilkins, pp. 1059–1094.

—— (1960), The mind-body relationship. In: *An Outline of Man's Knowledge of the Modern World*, ed. L. Bryson. New York: McGraw-Hill, pp. 41–72.

Zaiman, H., Frierson, J. G., & Shorter, R. G. (1988), Clinical aspects of certain parasitic infections affecting the large bowel in humans. In: *Diseases of the Colon, Rectum and Anal Canal*, ed. J. B. Kirsner & R. G. Shorter. Baltimore: Williams & Wilkins, pp. 483–506.

Zetzel, E. R. (1956), Current concepts of transference. *Internat. J. Psycho-Anal.*, 37:369–376.

Name Index

261

Subject Index

267